Technology and Big Data in Rheumatology

Editors

JEFFREY R. CURTIS
KALEB MICHAUD
KEVIN WINTHROP

RHEUMATIC DISEASE CLINICS OF NORTH AMERICA

www.rheumatic.theclinics.com

Consulting Editor
MICHAEL H. WEISMAN

May 2019 • Volume 45 • Number 2

ELSEVIER

1600 John F. Kennedy Boulevard • Suite 1800 • Philadelphia, Pennsylvania, 19103-2899

http://www.theclinics.com

RHEUMATIC DISEASE CLINICS OF NORTH AMERICA Volume 45, Number 2

May 2019 ISSN 0889-857X, ISBN 13: 978-0-323-67862-9

Editor: Lauren Boyle
Developmental Editor: Casey Potter

Rheumatic Disease Clinics of North America (ISSN 0889-857X) is published quarterly by Elsevier Inc., 360 Park Avenue South, New York, NY 10010-1710. Months of issue are February, May, August, and November. Business and editorial offices: 1600 John F. Kennedy Boulevard, Suite 1800, Philadelphia, PA 19103-2899. Periodicals postage paid at New York, NY and additional mailing offices. Subscription prices are USD 362.00 per year for US individuals, USD 706.00 per year for US institutions, USD 100.00 per year for US students and residents, USD 427.00 per year for Canadian individuals, USD 925.00 per year for Canadian institutions, USD 465.00 per year for international individuals, USD 925.00 per year for international institutions, and USD 230.00 per year for Canadian and foreign students/residents. To receive student/resident rate, orders must be accompanied by name of affiliated institution, date of term, and the *signature* of program/residency coordinator on institution letterhead. Orders will be billed at individual rate until proof of status received. Foreign air speed delivery is included in all *Clinics* subscription prices. All prices are subject to change without notice. **POSTMASTER:** Send address changes to *Rheumatic Disease Clinics of North America,* Elsevier Health Sciences Division, Subscription Customer Service, 3251 Riverport Lane, Maryland Heights, MO 63043. **Customer Service: 1-800-654-2452 (US and Canada). From outside of the US and Canada: 314-447-8871. Fax: 314-447-8029. For print support, e-mail: JournalsCustomerService-usa@elsevier.com**. **For online support, e-mail: JournalsOnline Support-usa@elsevier.com**.

Reprints. For copies of 100 or more of articles in this publication, please contact the Commercial Reprints Department, Elsevier Inc., 360 Park Avenue South, New York, New York, 10010-1710; Tel.: +1-212-633-3874, Fax: +1-212-633-3820, and E-mail: reprints@elsevier.com.

Rheumatic Disease Clinics of North America is covered in *MEDLINE/PubMed (Index Medicus), Current Contents/Clinical Medicine, Science Citation Index, ISI/BIOMED,* and *EMBASE/Excerpta Medica.*

Contributors

CONSULTING EDITOR

MICHAEL H. WEISMAN, MD
Cedars-Sinai Chair in Rheumatology, Director, Division of Rheumatology, Professor of Medicine Emeritus, Cedars-Sinai Medical Center, Distinguished Professor of Medicine Emeritus, David Geffen School of Medicine at UCLA, Los Angeles, California, USA

EDITORS

JEFFREY R. CURTIS, MD, MS, MPH
Harbart Ball Professor of Medicine, Division of Clinical Immunology and Rheumatology, The University of Alabama at Birmingham, Birmingham, Alabama, USA

KALEB MICHAUD, PhD
Associate Professor, Division of Rheumatology and Immunology, University of Nebraska Medical Center, Omaha, Nebraska, USA; Co-Director, FORWARD, The National Databank for Rheumatic Diseases, Wichita, Kansas, USA

KEVIN WINTHROP, MD, MPH
Professor, Division of Infectious Diseases, Oregon Health & Sciences University, Portland, Oregon, USA

AUTHORS

METTE AADAHL, PT, MPH, PhD
Associate Professor, Centre for Clinical Research and Prevention, Bispebjerg and Frederiksberg Hospital, Frederiksberg, Denmark; Department of Public Health, Faculty of Health and Medical Sciences, University of Copenhagen, Copenhagen, Denmark

PAUL BIRD, PhD, GradDipMRI, FRACP
University of New South Wales, Kogarah, Sydney, New South Wales, Australia

VIVIAN P. BYKERK, MD, FRCPC
Director of the Inflammatory Arthritis Center, Division of Rheumatology, Hospital for Special Surgery, Associate Professor of Medicine, Weill Cornell Medical College, New York, New York, USA

DAVID CURTIS
Global Healthy Living Foundation, Upper Nyack, New York, USA

JEFFREY R. CURTIS, MD, MS, MPH
Harbart Ball Professor of Medicine, Division of Clinical Immunology and Rheumatology, The University of Alabama at Birmingham, Birmingham, Alabama, USA

WILLIAM G. DIXON, MRCP, PhD
Chair in Digital Epidemiology, Arthritis Research UK Centre for Epidemiology, University of Manchester, NIHR Manchester Musculoskeletal Biomedical Research Unit, Central Manchester University Hospitals NHS Foundation Trust, Manchester, United Kingdom

KATIE L. DRUCE, PhD
Research Associate, Arthritis Research UK Centre for Epidemiology, University of Manchester, Manchester, United Kingdom

BENTE APPEL ESBENSEN, RN, MSciN, PhD
Associate Professor, Research Manager, Copenhagen Center for Arthritis Research, Center for Rheumatology and Spine Diseases, Centre for Head and Orthopaedics, Rigshospitalet, Glostrup, Denmark; Department of Clinical Medicine, Faculty of Health and Medical Sciences, University of Copenhagen, Copenhagen, Denmark

P. JEFF FOSTER, MPH
Division of Clinical Immunology and Rheumatology, The University of Alabama at Birmingham, Birmingham, Alabama, USA

JULIE GANDRUP, MD
Division of Rheumatology, University of California, San Francisco, San Francisco, California, USA

KELLY GAVIGAN, MPH
Global Healthy Living Foundation, Upper Nyack, New York, USA

SETH GINSBERG
Global Healthy Living Foundation, Upper Nyack, New York, USA

MERETE LUND HETLAND, MD, PhD, DMSc
Professor, Consultant in Rheumatology, Copenhagen Center for Arthritis Research, Center for Rheumatology and Spine Diseases, Centre for Head and Orthopaedics, Rigshospitalet, Glostrup, Denmark; Department of Clinical Medicine Faculty of Health and Medical Sciences, University of Copenhagen, Copenhagen, Denmark; The DANBIO Registry, Center for Rheumatology and Spine Diseases, Centre for Head and Orthopaedics, Rigshospitalet, Denmark

E. MICHAEL LEWIECKI, MD
Clinical Assistant Professor of Medicine, University of New Mexico Health Sciences Center Director, Bone Health TeleECHO, Director, New Mexico Clinical Research & Osteoporosis Center, Albuquerque, New Mexico, USA

MARIA A. LOPEZ-OLIVO, MD, PhD
Assistant Professor, Section of Rheumatology and Clinical Immunology, Department of General Internal Medicine, The University of Texas MD Anderson Cancer Center, Houston, Texas, USA

JOHN McBETH, PhD
Reader in Epidemiology, Arthritis Research UK Centre for Epidemiology, University of Manchester, NIHR Manchester Musculoskeletal Biomedical Research Unit, Central Manchester University Hospitals NHS Foundation Trust, Manchester, United Kingdom

KALEB MICHAUD, PhD
Associate Professor, Division of Rheumatology and Immunology, University of Nebraska Medical Center, Omaha, Nebraska, USA; Co-Director, FORWARD, The National Databank for Rheumatic Diseases, Wichita, Kansas, USA

ELIZABETH MOLLARD, PhD
Assistant Professor, College of Nursing, University of Nebraska Medical Center, Lincoln, Nebraska, USA

WILLIAM BENJAMIN NOWELL, PhD
Global Healthy Living Foundation, Upper Nyack, New York, USA

RACHELLE ROCHELLE, MPA
Clinic Operation Manager, Project ECHO, University of New Mexico Health Sciences Center, Albuquerque, New Mexico, USA

SANNE A.A. RONGEN-VAN DARTEL, PhD
Department of Rheumatology, Bernhoven, Uden, The Netherlands; Radboud University Medical Center, Radboud Institute for Health Sciences, Scientific Institute for Quality of Healthcare (IQ Healthcare), Nijmegen, The Netherlands

KENNETH G. SAAG, MD, MSc
Division of Clinical Immunology and Rheumatology, The University of Alabama at Birmingham, Birmingham, Alabama, USA

MARIA E. SUAREZ-ALMAZOR, MD, PhD
Professor, Chief, Section of Rheumatology and Clinical Immunology, Department of General Internal Medicine, The University of Texas MD Anderson Cancer Center, Houston, Texas, USA

MICHELLE THAI
Media Cause, San Francisco, California, USA

TANJA THOMSEN, OT, MScH, PhD
Postdoc, Copenhagen Center for Arthritis Research, Center for Rheumatology and Spine Diseases, Centre for Head and Orthopaedics, Rigshospitalet, Glostrup, Denmark

PIET L.C.M. VAN RIEL, MD, PhD
Department of Rheumatology, Bernhoven, Uden, The Netherlands; Radboud University Medical Center, Radboud Institute for Health Sciences, Scientific Institute for Quality of Healthcare (IQ Healthcare), Nijmegen, The Netherlands

SHILPA VENKATACHALAM, PhD
Global Healthy Living Foundation, Upper Nyack, New York, USA

CARINE VOGEL, RN
Department of Rheumatology, Bernhoven, Uden, The Netherlands

CAROLE WIEDMEYER
Global Healthy Living Foundation, Upper Nyack, New York, USA

JINOOS YAZDANY, MD, MPH
Division of Rheumatology, University of California, San Francisco, San Francisco, California, USA

RIXT M. ZUIDEMA, MSc
Department of Rheumatology, Bernhoven, Uden, The Netherlands

Contents

Foreword: Technology and Big Data in Rheumatology xiii

Michael H. Weisman

Preface: The Interface Between Digital Health and Rheumatology xv

Jeffrey R. Curtis, Kaleb Michaud and Kevin Winthrop

Maximizing Engagement in Mobile Health Studies: Lessons Learned and Future Directions 159

Katie L. Druce, William G. Dixon, and John McBeth

The widespread availability of smartphones, tablets, and smartwatches has led to exponential growth in the number of mobile health (mHealth) studies conducted. Although promising, the key challenge of all apps (both for research and nonresearch) is the high attrition rate of participants and users. Numerous factors have been identified as potentially influencing engagement, and it is important that researchers consider these and how best to overcome them within their studies. This article discusses lessons learned from attempting to maximize engagement in 2 successful UK mHealth studies—Cloudy with a Chance of Pain and Quality of Life, Sleep and Rheumatoid Arthritis.

Digital Interventions to Build a Patient Registry for Rheumatology Research 173

William Benjamin Nowell, David Curtis, Michelle Thai, Carole Wiedmeyer, Kelly Gavigan, Shilpa Venkatachalam, Seth Ginsberg, and Jeffrey R. Curtis

This article aims to describe key issues, processes, and outcomes related to development of a patient registry for rheumatology research using a digital platform where patients track useful data about their condition for their own use while contributing to research. Digital interventions are effective to build a patient research registry for people with rheumatoid arthritis and other rheumatic and musculoskeletal diseases. ArthritisPower provides evidence of the value of digital interventions to build community support for research and to transform patient engagement and patient-generated data capture.

Patient Self-Management and Tracking: A European Experience 187

Piet L.C.M. van Riel, Rixt M. Zuidema, Carine Vogel, and Sanne A.A. Rongen-van Dartel

The shift from a paternalistic model of health care to a doctor-patient relationship in which the doctor and patient make shared decisions, requires an actively involved patient who takes responsibilities. This is why self-management by the patient with a chronic disease plays more of an important role in patient care nowadays; however, the degree of self-management varies per patient. To help stimulate patients in their self-management behavior, it is necessary to use an adequate tool, and to educate patients and health professionals. In this article, we share experiences using a digital tool for this from the Netherlands.

Mobile Apps for Rheumatoid Arthritis: Opportunities and Challenges **197**

Elizabeth Mollard and Kaleb Michaud

Mobile applications have the potential to improve health outcomes in patients with rheumatoid arthritis (RA). Whereas other chronic diseases such as diabetes and heart failure have a well-established presence in the mobile application realm, apps focused on RA are still in their infancy. This article presents an overview of the types of mobile apps that can be used for RA and discusses the opportunities and challenges associated with them.

Patient-Reported Outcomes Measurement Information System Versus Legacy Instruments: Are They Ready for Prime Time? **211**

Vivian P. Bykerk

"Legacy" patient-reported outcome measures (PROs) have been used for decades; however, they have many limitations. The National Institutes of Health–funded PRO Measurement Information System (PROMIS) was developed to be a generic, flexible, precise, and reliable tool to measure core and additional domains of physical and emotional health and social well-being. Unlike Legacy PROs, PROMIS measures can be implemented across diseases, and use a common T-score metric-based scoring system derived using item response theory. PROMIS measure scores have potential to predict scores of Legacy PROs and could be the only set of measures needed to assess PROs.

Motivational Counseling and Text Message Reminders: For Reduction of Daily Sitting Time and Promotion of Everyday Physical Activity in People with Rheumatoid Arthritis **231**

Tanja Thomsen, Bente Appel Esbensen, Merete Lund Hetland, and Mette Aadahl

Most patients with rheumatoid arthritis tend to be physically inactive and spend more time in sedentary behaviors compared with the general population. This inactive lifestyle can lead to serious health consequences, for example, increased risk of cardiovascular disease. For this reason, there is an interest in increasing participation in physical activity in patients with rheumatoid arthritis. The relatively new approach of reducing sedentary behavior and replacing it with light-intensity physical activity has been shown to be feasible and effective in promoting physical activity in patients with rheumatoid arthritis. However, methods to facilitate this behavior have not yet been fully explored.

Digital Patient Education and Decision Aids **245**

Maria A. Lopez-Olivo and Maria E. Suarez-Almazor

New technologies can do more than just digitize health information; they can support multimedia platforms for patient education and health decision support. Technology can simplify the way health decisions are made by offering quick access to a vast amount of information that can be tailored to specific populations. Digital tools can increase knowledge and assist consumers in comparing health care alternatives. They are well received by patients because of the myriad features that render them visually appealing and entertaining, including audiovisual and interactive elements. To be effective, however, digital tools must be evidence based and developed following quality standards.

Using Health Information Technology to Support Use of Patient-Reported Outcomes in Rheumatology **257**

Julie Gandrup and Jinoos Yazdany

Technology can help health care providers understand their patients' experience of illness in a way that was previously impossible. Experience in using health information technology (IT) to capture this information through PROs within rheumatology suggests that careful attention to human centered design, including detailed workflow planning, consideration of patient and physician burden, integration into the health IT ecosystem, and delivering information to the right person at the right time are all important. Technology applications must be tested in diverse health systems and populations to ensure they are simple to interpret, useful for clinical decision making and effective in impacting outcomes.

Tools and Methods for Real-World Evidence Generation: Pragmatic Trials, Electronic Consent, and Data Linkages **275**

Jeffrey R. Curtis, P. Jeff Foster, and Kenneth G. Saag

Real-world evidence requires use of new tools and methods to support efficient evidence generation. Among those tools are pragmatic trials, utilization of central/single institutional review board and electronic consent, and data linkages between diverse types of data sources (eg, a trial or registry to administrative claims or electronic medical record data). This article reviews these topics in the context of describing several exemplar use cases specific to rheumatology and provides perspective regarding both the promise and potential pitfalls in using these tools and approaches.

Imaging in the Mobile Domain **291**

Paul Bird

This article outlines the current state of imaging software with an emphasis on mobile sharing of images and mobile sharing of imaged data. The second portion focuses on the mobility of imaging design devices, highlighting the accessibility and the wider application of mobile devices.

Project ECHO: Telehealth to Expand Capacity to Deliver Best Practice Medical Care **303**

E. Michael Lewiecki and Rachelle Rochelle

Project ECHO (Extension for Community Healthcare Outcomes) was developed at the University of New Mexico Health Sciences Center to educate health care professionals in underserved communities to treat chronic complex diseases, allowing patients to receive better care, closer to home, with greater convenience, and at lower cost than referral to a specialty center. Videoconferencing technology is used to create learning networks, with case-based discussions as the primary method of education. The 3-year experience of Bone Health TeleECHO, a strategy to improve the care of osteoporosis and reduce the large treatment gap, is discussed.

RHEUMATIC DISEASE CLINICS OF NORTH AMERICA

FORTHCOMING ISSUES

August 2019
Controversies in Rheumatology
John Kay and Sergio Schwartzman, *Editors*

November 2019
Treat to Target in Rheumatic Diseases: Rationale and Results
Daniel Aletaha, *Editor*

February 2020
Education and Professional Development in Rheumatology
James Katz and Karina Torralba, *Editors*

RECENT ISSUES

February 2019
Best Practices and Challenges to the Practice of Rheumatology
Daniel J. Wallace and Swamy Venuturupalli, *Editors*

November 2018
Renal Involvement in Rheumatic Diseases
Andrew Bomback and Meghan E. Sise, *Editors*

August 2018
Medical Practice Challenges for the Rheumatologist
James D. Katz and Brian Walitt, *Editors*

SERIES OF RELATED INTEREST

Physical Medicine and Rehabilitation Clinics
https://www.pmr.theclinics.com/
Medical Clinics
https://www.medical.theclinics.com/
Primary Care Clinics
https://www.primarycare.theclinics.com/
Dermatologic Clinics
https://www.derm.theclinics.com/

THE CLINICS ARE AVAILABLE ONLINE!
Access your subscription at:
www.theclinics.com

Foreword

Technology and Big Data in Rheumatology

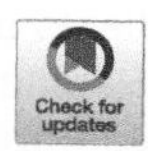

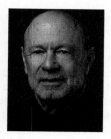

Michael H. Weisman, MD
Consulting Editor

This issue was intended to examine the impact of new technology and "big data" on the field of Rheumatology, and it certainly met its goals. Drs Winthrop, Curtis, and Michaud have assembled very thoughtful and incisive pieces to address how, if, or why these "new tools" will have an impact on our research, education, and practice effort in Rheumatology.

Drs Lopez-Olivo and Suarez-Almazor, in an outstanding contribution, discuss the important distinction between health information and health education, emphasizing the complexity of health education that necessarily involves making sure that it contains accurate information with the best evidence possible along with a clear understanding on how to maintain personal health. Assessing the value of digital patient education and decision aids must be placed in this context since rheumatic conditions are complex both cognitively and emotionally. Professor Paul Bird discusses the state-of-the-art as well as the future of mobile sharing of images and imaged data. He describes the currently available tools for image transfer, display, and interpretation as well as the future for the use of portable and accessible ultrasound, MRI, and artificial intelligence in radiology. The future appears to be unbelievably robust. However, a different message is delivered by Druce, Dixon, and McBeth as they examine the widespread availability of smartphones, tablets, and apps in epidemiologic research. The message here is how to address the challenge of the high attrition rate of participants and users. Gandrup and Yazdany address the increasing application of electronic PRO collections as a tool for health care planning and research; they emphasize the need to understand both providers and patients' perspectives. However, their own experience and the literature suggest that issues need to be addressed, such as human-centered design, workflow planning, and patient and physician burden. They point out that for this new technology to achieve its goals it must be tested in diverse patient populations.

Rheum Dis Clin N Am 45 (2019) xiii–xiv
https://doi.org/10.1016/j.rdc.2019.02.002

Van Riel and colleagues describe the European experience with self-management of Rheumatoid Arthritis, where they have developed a digital tool to educate both patients and health professionals. Although it is uniquely European in its approach, the ReumaNet tool along with the commitment of van Riel and his group is an excellent example of how a patient can monitor and manage their disease outcome in the modern technology world. Thomsen and colleagues address, through digital technology approaches, the positive outcome of reducing the inactive and sedentary behavior of rheumatoid arthritis patients that if left alone would result in adverse health outcomes. A remarkable platform using digital interventions to build a patient registry for research has been accomplished and is now described by Nowell and colleagues, but it is important to acknowledge the steps, problems, and pitfalls for doing so successfully. Long-term engagement to a patient community without prior research ties is the most effective approach, and regular touch points with participants are critical for long-term success. Drs Lewiecki and Rochelle describe Project ECHO using videoconferencing technology that creates learning networks with case-based discussions as the primary method of education. Although designed to educate health care professionals in underserved areas, this approach can be utilized to reduce treatment gaps for delivering specialty care in a variety of settings. Drs Curtis, Foster, and Saag approach the evidence gap in medical practice by addressing the values (and pitfalls) of obtaining real-world evidence from new tools, such as pragmatic trials, technology-based methods that facilitate electronic consent, and new methods of linkages between disparate data sources to answer research questions. Mollard and Michaud also address the issue of mobile technology by focusing on its use and implementation in Rheumatoid Arthritis. There are opportunities as well as challenges to this approach of accumulating objective information; however, despite the initial enthusiasm that was generated when these methods arrived on the scene, there are real concerns about the limited evidence for their ability to improve outcomes and to overcome both patient and provider barriers in Rheumatoid Arthritis. Finally, Dr Vivien Bykerk in a thoughtful analysis discusses the evolution of health status measurement tools from the legacy instruments to the now widely adopted technology-advanced PROMIS tool. She emphasizes that more work needs to be done in the implementation sphere since simply incorporating these measures into the electronic health record is not sufficient to ensure that they are used in a meaningful way.

Michael H. Weisman, MD
Division of Rheumatology
Cedars-Sinai Medical Center
David Geffen School of Medicine at UCLA
1545 Calmar Court
Los Angeles, CA 90024, USA

E-mail address:
Michael.Weisman@csh.org

Preface

The Interface Between Digital Health and Rheumatology

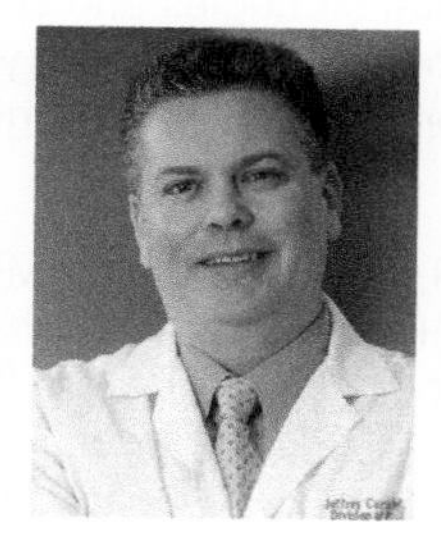

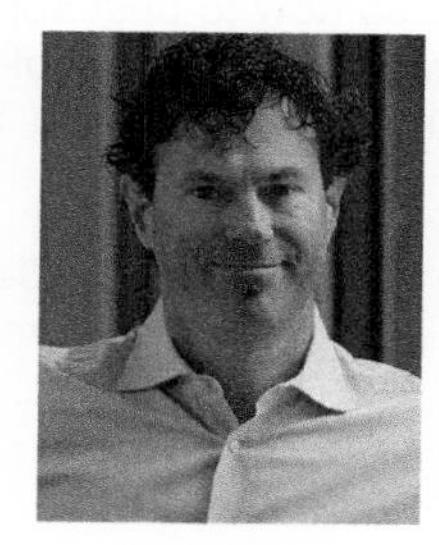

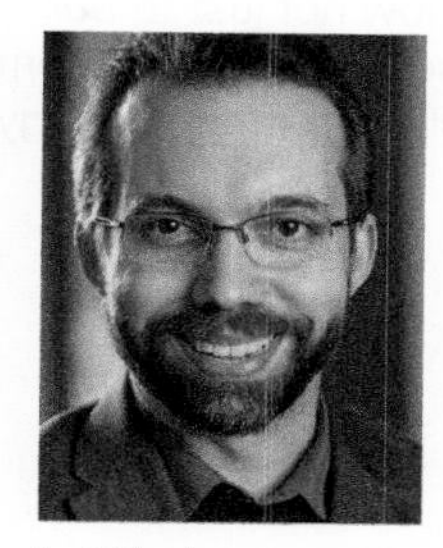

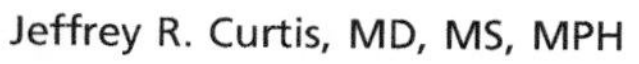

Jeffrey R. Curtis, MD, MS, MPH   Kaleb Michaud, PhD   Kevin Winthrop, MD, MPH
Editors

Technology is effecting a sea of change in both health care research and the practice of clinical medicine. In this technology-focused issue of *Rheumatic Disease Clinics of North America*, we have assembled a cadre of reports that illustrate the wide breadth of examples by which technology is transforming both research methods and clinical practice in rheumatology. Many of these articles were borne out of presentations given at the 2018 American College of Rheumatology (ACR) premeeting clinical research conference (CRC), "Application of Mobile Health Technologies." The ACR and its membership continue to maintain high interest in digital health, as illustrated by the fact that the 2019 ACR preconference CRC topic is "Big Data: Analytics, Electronic Medical Records, Registries, and Beyond."

The topics included in this issue span novel (but practical) methods to digitally capture patient-reported outcomes in real-world settings and make the data interpretable and actionable to both patients and clinicians; digitally administered education and behavioral interventions for arthritis patients; and methods to support pragmatic trials and data linkages, capture, and process image data, and facilitate telemedicine approaches to care delivery.

Despite the tremendous buzz and enthusiasm surrounding digital health, several misconceptions must be dispelled. Perhaps the most important of these is the notion that the problems to be addressed, and the possible solutions to be created, are mostly technical in nature. Indeed, one might naively believe that better uptake of smartphone apps, cloud-based data storage with improved electronic interfaces and secure data-sharing methods, advanced analytics (including machine learning and artificial intelligence), and a more robust mobile digital infrastructure (including the Internet of Things), will yield the expected efficiencies already being enjoyed by consumers and by the business world. In fact, this is unlikely to be the case. A number of recent examples of technology applied to medicine (including rheumatology)[1,2]

Rheum Dis Clin N Am 45 (2019) xv–xvi
https://doi.org/10.1016/j.rdc.2019.02.001

illustrate the familiar "technology hype cycle"[3] whereby we travel from the peak of inflated initial expectations and into the trough of disillusionment. Only by recognizing what we don't know can we then start to ascend the slope of enlightenment.

Technology is like any other tool, and by itself, is necessary but not sufficient to advance research and improve medical care. For that reason, problems that might heretofore have been seen as technical in nature are becoming increasingly recognized as social and behavioral challenges. Medicine is on a transformative journey to learn how not just to build, but also how to best apply, digital strategies and solutions to solve today's and tomorrow's health care problems. To that end, we invite you to sample the rheumatology-focused topics in this burgeoning domain of digital health.

Jeffrey R. Curtis, MD, MS, MPH
University of Alabama at Birmingham
Faculty Office Towers 802
510 20th Street South
Birmingham, AL 35294, USA

Kaleb Michaud, PhD
University of Nebraska Medical Center
FORWARD
The National Databank for Rheumatic Diseases
986270 Nebraska Medical Center
Omaha, NE 68198-6270, USA

Kevin Winthrop, MD, MPH
Division of Infectious Diseases
Oregon Health and Sciences University
3181 SW Sam Jackson Park Road
Mail Code GH104
Portland, OR 97239-3098, USA

E-mail addresses:
jrcurtis@uabmc.edu (J.R. Curtis)
kmichaud@unmc.edu (K. Michaud)
winthrop@ohsu.edu (K. Winthrop)

REFERENCES

1. Proffitt, A. What GlaxoSmithKline Learned From Their Digital Trial of Rheumatoid Arthritis; 2019. Available at: http://www.clinicalinformaticsnews.com/2018/03/08/what-glaxosmithkline-learned-from-their-digital-trial-rheumatoid-arthritis.aspx. Accessed February 12, 2019.
2. Pevnick JM, Fuller G, Duncan R, et al. A Large-Scale Initiative Inviting Patients to Share Personal Fitness Tracker Data with Their Providers: Initial Results. PLoS One 2016;11(11):e0165908. Available at: https://www.ncbi.nlm.nih.gov/pmc/articles/PMC5112984. Accessed February 12, 2019.
3. Hype Cycle Research Methodology. 2019. Available at: https://www.gartner.com/en/research/methodologies/gartner-hype-cycle. Accessed February 12, 2019.

Maximizing Engagement in Mobile Health Studies

Lessons Learned and Future Directions

Katie L. Druce, PhD[a,*], William G. Dixon, MRCP, PhD[a,b], John McBeth, PhD[a,b]

KEYWORDS

- Epidemiology • mHealth • Methods • Remote monitoring • Rheumatic diseases
- Patient reported outcomes

KEY POINTS

- The widespread availability of smartphones, tablets, and apps presents an exciting opportunity for epidemiologic research.
- Although promising, the key challenge of all apps (both for research and nonresearch) is the high attrition rate of participants and users.
- Any engagement strategies used should consider usability of technology, push or motivating factors, and the need for personal contact with study personnel (not just technology) and study support.
- Particular benefits to long-term engagement may occur through the use of real-time data monitoring and passive monitoring and by providing personalized study feedback.
- Future studies should consider adopting and advancing these approaches at an early stage of study design to maximize patient engagement.

INTRODUCTION

The Promise of Apps to Support Data Collection for Health Research

The widespread availability of smartphones, tablets, and smartwatches and common usage of apps,[1,2] particularly for health care monitoring,[3,4] present an exciting opportunity for epidemiologic research to reach and recruit high proportions of the population. Furthermore, using apps and other mobile health (mHealth) technology, such as wearables, researchers can now conduct frequent and repeated remote collection of self-report data, such as symptom reports, and objective assessments of biometrics (eg, heart rate), sleep, physical activity, and active tasks, such as walking tasks to

Disclosure Statement: The authors have nothing to disclose.
[a] Arthritis Research UK Centre for Epidemiology, University of Manchester, Manchester, UK;
[b] NIHR Manchester Musculoskeletal Biomedical Research Unit, Central Manchester University Hospitals NHS Foundation Trust, Manchester, UK
* Corresponding author.
E-mail address: Katie.druce@manchester.ac.uk

Rheum Dis Clin N Am 45 (2019) 159–172
https://doi.org/10.1016/j.rdc.2019.01.004 **rheumatic.theclinics.com**
0889-857X/19/

determine gait and balance.[5–8] mHealth studies can thus increasingly provide data to investigate day-to-day patterns of disease and embed objective markers of symptom and disease factors through time more readily than traditional models (eg, registries), which tend to investigate change between disparate time points (eg, every 6–12 months).

The Challenge of Maintaining Engagement

Although promising, a fundamental challenge for those seeking to conduct app studies is the seemingly ubiquitous phenomenon of rapid and substantial disengagement from apps[9] for both research and nonresearch. For example, despite one of the most successful smartphone games of recent years, Pokémon Go (https://pokemongolive.com/en/) experienced a loss of one-third (15 million) of their daily active users within 1 month of the launch date.[10] Estimates indicate that approximately 71% of app users across all industries (eg, media and entertainment, retail, lifestyle, and business) disengage within 90 days[11]; in health research studies, as few as approximately 10% to 25% of recruited participants have been shown engaged in studies by the end of data-entry protocols that collect data from once per week to 3 times a day, lasting between 1 week and 12 weeks.[5,12,13]

Among research studies, loss of engagement can have substantial impacts on the integrity of data collected within mHealth studies, creating issues, such as bias (if those who disengage are systematically different from those who do not), reduced data quality, and high rates of data missingness. Furthermore, lack of transparency in study design or reporting can lead to misinterpretation if it is not clear how many people entered and remained in a study and what the factors are that drive that engagement. Failure to address or prevent these threats may mean that mHealth studies produce incorrect conclusions about the existence, strength, or direction of associations between exposures and outcomes.[14]

For those seeking to overcome these challenges, the importance of maximizing participant engagement is paramount. Insights also may be obtained from reflecting on the design and engagement processes used in other successful mHealth studies.

The Success of Apps

Two recently completed mHealth studies conducted within the Arthritis Research UK Centre for Epidemiology at the University of Manchester have had notable success with respect to recruiting and engaging participants for between 30 days and 12 months.

The first study, Cloudy with a Chance of Pain,[15,16] is a UK smartphone-based study that sought to examine the link between the weather and pain in people with chronic pain. Participants were recruited to the study using a variety of advertisements both in mainstream and social media. Importantly, participants had no contact with the research team prior to registration and instead accessed the study Web site, self-downloaded the app, and registered remotely. After registration, participants were asked to complete a baseline questionnaire and report symptoms once per day (estimated 1–2 minutes per entry) for 6 months (latterly extended to 12 months). Meanwhile, the smartphone's Global Positioning System (GPS) reported hourly location, allowing linkage to local weather data from the Met Office (the UK national weather service). The authors demonstrated that approximately 1 in 7 participants were highly engaged for 6 months in a study investigating whether self-reported pain severity is associated with weather variables, completing full data entry on 89% of all possible days.[15]

The second study, Quality of Life, Sleep and Rheumatoid Arthritis (QUASAR), examined the relationship between sleep and quality of life among people with rheumatoid arthritis. Participants were recruited through advertisements disseminated by the UK National Rheumatoid Arthritis Society and displayed in several National Health Service secondary care clinics (or rheumatology offices) and primary care surgeries (or doctors' offices). Potential participants completed an online screening questionnaire and were recruited directly by the study team during recruitment telephone calls. After completion of a baseline questionnaire, digital data collection comprised a morning daily sleep diary and symptom assessment (estimated 5–7 minutes of data entry) and an evening symptom assessment (estimated 1–2 minutes of data entry) for 30 days and a series of follow-up questionnaires on days 10, 20, 30, and 60 of the study. During the 30 days of continuous symptom monitoring, participants were also asked to wear a triaxial accelerometer to continuously record daytime activity and estimate evening sleep parameters. Of 285 participants recruited, 270 participants could be included in the study (gave full consent and successfully returned the study pack). In total, 91% (n = 246) of participants met the reporting criteria necessary to be defined as an engaged user over the 1-month study period (at least 15/30 days of symptoms and sleep diary and 2/4 follow-up questionnaires).

The success of these studies is due to the considered strategies used to maximize participant engagement, including focusing on usability of technology, functional ability of participants, and consideration of participant workload and time commitment; push or motivating factors, such as the use of reminders; data monitoring; provision of study contact details; and study support. This article describes the strategies used and lessons learned. It uses participant quotations (provided in participant e-mails, via social media, or in response to formal feedback requests) to highlight how successful the strategies were in promoting engagement.

PATIENT ADVISORY GROUPS

First and foremost, it is important to consider the use of patient advisory groups (PAGs), who are well positioned to codesign the study by identifying potential barriers for participants and help craft possible solutions. Members of any PAG developed should comprise people who have lived experience with the condition or symptom of interest in the study. Ideally, participants have a range of levels of disease severity and experience with both technology and research more generally.

The authors' PAGs comprised volunteers from the Greater Manchester, UK, area with chronic pain (Cloudy with a Chance of Pain) or rheumatoid arthritis (RA) (QUASAR), who responded to requests for participants disseminated through the University of Manchester Centre for Musculoskeletal Research User Group online support networks or social media. Participants had a range of experience with technology and included active smartphone users and individuals who had never used a smartphone. Most participants had some experience in research, although not specifically in research using digital data collection. PAG members were asked to discuss various aspects of study designs, including the frequency and content of data collection, and to identify any barriers or facilitators to participation in studies using digital data collection.

USABILITY OF TECHNOLOGY—FUNCTIONAL ABILITY AND WORKLOAD AND TIME REQUIRED

Functional Ability of the Study Population

Attrition is likely higher among people who experience functional/logistical limitations using the app. Thus, specific considerations must be given to the suitability of the devices provided for the target population. For example, the sleep monitor used with the

QUASAR study has an event marker, which participants were asked to use to indicate when they got in and out of bed. The authors, however, had numerous reports from participants that they had difficulty with the monitor due to issues of dexterity and hand function:

I have put the monitor on this morning, and touched the centre disc I don't have very good sensitivity in my fingers, so wonder if you can check your end that I am applying enough pressure.

—QUASAR participant

I have attempted to press the button...but I have no sense as to whether I am meant to feel the button depress...This may be because the fingers on my right hand are quite swollen and lack much feeling at the tips.

—QUASAR participant

In one instance, a participant came up with the solution to use a stylus used for their other devices and was able to successfully use the marker thereafter. Many participants stopped using the marker, instead focusing on completing the morning sleep diary to report the previous night's sleep period. This issue was not noted within the QUASAR PAGs, which comprised patients with RA discussing aspects of the study design, or by the healthy volunteer pilot testers who wore the monitor for 7 days. The authors noted, however, that the monitor was extensively worn only by healthy volunteer testers and it may have been that this issue would have been highlighted if members of the PAGs had instead worn the monitor for the 7-day pilot study. Thus, despite the usefulness of the PAGs and piloting in identifying several key barriers and facilitators for participation in the study, these processes were not sufficient. In future, where a study requires the use of new or unfamiliar technology, it would be beneficial to conduct extensive patient piloting in the initial stages of study design and pilot test implementation.

Workload and Time Required

Although some degree of attrition is inevitable in longitudinal research, it is likely that the attrition is greater and more rapid when participant burden (both in terms of frequency and complexity of data collection) is higher.[9,17] Yet, data collection for comprehensive mHealth studies must include the collection of data on all relevant exposures, outcomes, and putative confounders and may become particularly burdensome when all 3 variable types are time varying (ie, their values change over time.)[18]

It is essential that the study design considers the most parsimonious data collection protocol possible from a participant's point of view, while being sufficiently comprehensive to collect all data necessary. The authors recommend that to optimize data collection, researchers should codesign their study with PAGs, thus gathering a range of opinions from individuals on the amount, frequency, timing, and type of data collection that can be best integrated into daily life. For example, the authors' PAGs determined that it would be acceptable to report data at 1 time point per day for 6 months (latterly extended to 1 year [Cloudy with a Chance of Pain]) and twice per day for 1 month (QUASAR). In discussing the frequency of data collection per day, the authors were able to create data collection protocols, which participants found well suited to their lives:

It's all very easy and straightforward to do every day.

—Cloudy with a Chance of Pain participant

It's become a habit now, part of the routine of the day.

—Cloudy with a Chance of Pain participant

App is simple to use. Very convenient.

—*QUASAR participant*

Happy to partake in any studies that provide research into RA and don't drastically disrupt my life!

—*QUASAR participant*

The perceived ease of use is largely due to the core uMotif platform used across both studies that comprises a simple graphical interface (**Fig. 1**) and is attractive to users and quick to complete (estimated 1–2 minutes per entry).[6,16] The uMotif interface comprises 10 segments, each of which represents a symptom that can be moved to give an ordinal 5-point outcome (eg, pain severity measured as 1 "no pain" to 5 "very severe pain"). Participants tap each of the 10 segments to highlight the relevant symptom and move the colored section to denote symptom severity.

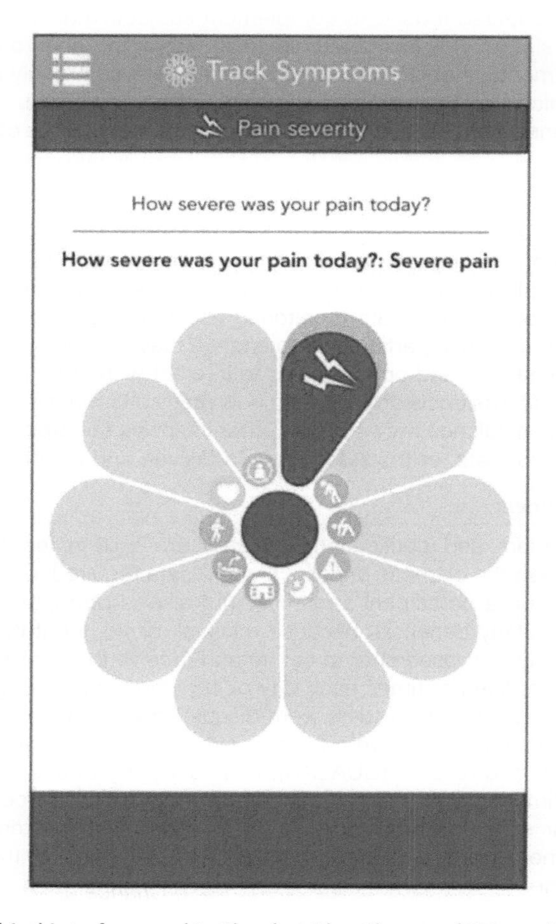

Fig. 1. Main graphical interface used in Cloudy with a Chance of Pain and QUASAR. Each of the 10 segments represents a different symptom, such as pain severity (highlighted), measured on a 5-point ordinal scale.

Participant burden may be reduced further by the use of passive monitoring. Passive monitoring is defined as a data collection technique that can collect relevant information without active engagement from the participant. Techniques may include the use of physical activity monitors (eg, accelerometers), heart rate or blood pressure monitors, or other built-in features of the mHealth device, such as gyroscopes.[6,19,20,21] In the authors' studies, the built-in GPS tracking on participants' smartphones (Cloudy with a Chance of Pain) and sleep monitors (QUASAR) was used to capture data passively. The authors have found that such methods of data collection are acceptable to participants providing they do not experience a reduction in the battery life of their devices (eg, GPS) or that any wearable technology (eg, sleep monitors) is discreet and unobtrusive. No privacy issues were raised with respect to the collection of geolocation, although it is not known whether any potential participants were put off of participating in the Cloudy with a Chance of Pain study due to concerns of privacy.

Embedding passive monitoring within studies not only may enable improved engagement and reduced participant burden but also may give greater dimensionality to the data collected if used to complement subjective assessments, such as when measuring sleep.[6] This increased dimensionality may serve to improve the accuracy of assessments, if objective markers can replace commonly used subjective assessments, which may be subject to reporting errors and biases. Although promising, there remains a need to validate and standardize many of the objective outputs available.

PUSH FACTORS

Push factors to promote engagement may range from generic strategies, such as the use of automatic daily prompts or alerts for data completion, to a more intensive and bespoke process of real-time data monitoring and targeted completion reminders. Other factors that may push participants to engage may include ongoing study feedback, networking effects, and opportunities to interact with other participants within study communities.[9] The decision regarding how many different types of push factors to use, however, is a balance between how labor intensive the processes are for software developers to create, or the study team to deliver, and the benefits received.

Automated Reminders

Automated reminders and notifications typically are built-in features of mHealth studies and increase the chances of collecting the data required, because data entry not only is reliant on a participant's memory but also is prompted. Automated reminders are particularly beneficial because minimal, or no, input is required on the part of the participant or researcher to set up and receive the reminders. Reminders may be delivered at fixed at times each day or semirandomly throughout the day.[19] Within the authors' studies, reminders were discussed within the relevant PAGs and agreed suitable reminder times were fixed at either 6.24 PM (Cloudy with a Chance of Pain) or 8.00 AM and 6.00 PM (QUASAR). It is necessary to use caution, however, in deciding the timeframe in which reminders are sent because certain times may be unsuitable for specific participants, such as those who are employed in shift work (who were necessarily excluded from the QUASAR study) or those who have a fixed social routine:

> *I have quite a busy life and go swimming early most mornings then sometimes I forget if I have entered my symptoms.*
>
> *—QUASAR participant*

Is it possible to change the times for the reminders? Now I've done it a couple of times I realise they're not quite right for me at the moment. I'd ideally like them at 7:30 and 18:30.

—QUASAR participant

For future studies, it may be worth considering whether it would be beneficial to allow participants to dictate the times at which they would like to receive their reminders, provided this flexibility has no detrimental impact on the exposures and outcomes under investigation (ie, neither factor is time-sensitive).

Real-time data monitoring and targeted completion reminders

If reminders are unsuccessful and participants have not completed data collection, it has been shown that real-time data monitoring and active chasing of participants (ie, sending targeted completion reminders) can be successful in preventing dropout and maximizing data completion.[9] This approach was adopted within the QUASAR study, with a data monitoring process was developed to identify participants at risk of disengagement and to send participants 1 of 3 noncompletion text messages, to encourage re-engagement and data completion.

Data monitoring was completed every second business day (Monday–Friday) after the manual download of data from the study portal created by uMotif to the research team data environment. An internally developed database script then analyzed the data download and alerted the study team (via e-mail) to any participants who had not completed symptom or sleep diary data for 3 days or who had not completed a follow-up as expected. On receiving the alert, the study team checked the report and confirmed that relevant participants should receive a text message to encourage completion (eg, **Fig. 2**). The study team could ensure that participants were not continually chased for data completion; instead, a maximum of 2 messages would be sent before a phone call was made to try to directly contact the participant and discuss any problems.

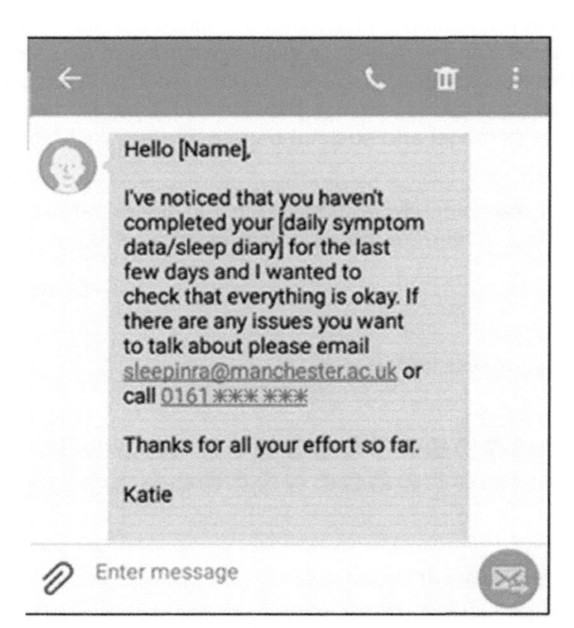

Fig. 2. Example of noncompletion reminder text message sent during the QUASAR study.

A total of 315 noncompletion messages were sent during the QUASAR study to 181 (63.5%) unique patients: 7 registrations not completed on the agreed study start day, 52 greater than or equal to 3 days of missing symptom or sleep diary data (14 symptoms and 38 sleep diaries), and 256 follow-up questionnaires not completed on the day expected. After these text messages, 3 registrations were completed (42%), 201 follow-up questionnaires were completed (79%), and 36 people recommenced frequent completion of sleep diary or symptom data (69%; example shown in **Fig. 3**). With the exception of the follow-up questionnaires, few people required repeated chasing to complete data entry. Just 3 people (1%) were contacted twice to prompt completion of sleep diaries or symptoms, whereas 49 people were contacted twice or more to complete follow-up questionnaires (eg, they had not completed their days 10 and 20 follow-ups). A total of 3 people (1%) were contacted for missingness of symptoms, sleep diaries, and at least 1 follow-up.

The application of such near real-time screening for data missingness is clearly beneficial, but, unless processes of data monitoring and text message creation are automated, the use of such strategies may be labor intensive for the research team. Thus, it is important to balance the effort likely to be expended with the achievable benefits (eg, the increase in amount of completed data or increased proportion of people meeting minimum data requirement). Rules also should be developed to agree to a reasonable time period, or frequency, with which participants can be prompted to provide data, without risking participants feeling harassed or coerced into providing data.

Personal Motivations

Individuals may be more likely to participate in studies of experiences that have affected them personally or in studies where they perceive a wider societal benefit.[22] Personal motivations for participating in studies were highlighted in PAGs held for both exemplar studies as being the desire to contribute to answering an understandable and engaging research question (Cloudy with a Chance of Pain) and due to personal experience of the poor management of an illness or symptom and desire to develop a suitable management solution (QUASAR). Importantly, by addressing a research question that is important or meaningful to the participants, their contribution is perceived of greater personal and societal benefit, thereby increasing the likelihood of engagement:

> *It's really good to see some in-depth research into sleep and RA... sleep is way more important than most of us give it credit for, and RA is no doubt extremely disruptive to it.*
>
> *—QUASAR participant*

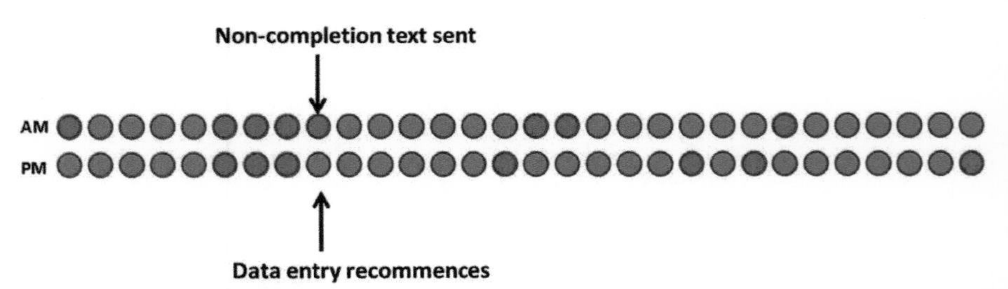

Fig. 3. Data-entry report for the QUASAR study, with notation for when noncompletion text was sent and data entry recommenced.

I personally am in no doubt the weather/pressure/temperature has a monumental effect on conditions of chronic pain and am very grateful that this study is being done, and that someone actually wants to research it and help
—Cloudy with a Chance of Pain participant

It is noteworthy that Cloudy with a Chance of Pain built on participants' desires to contribute to answering the research question by asking participants and the wider public to engage in a citizen science project (**Fig. 4**) to view and interact with the data collected during the study and submit new, or revised, hypotheses about the link between pain and the weather. A total of 418 hypotheses were submitted by both study participants and members of the wider public. Participants were also reminded that their ongoing data completion and engagement were valued in text messages (QUASAR), weekly newsletters (Cloudy with a Chance of Pain), and relevant study emails. As a result, participants were able to constantly see the benefits of ongoing data completion and were aware that their data are valuable and actively contributing to the researcher's ability to answer the studies aim.

Study Feedback

In addition to a desire to contribute data to address the research question, PAG members highlighted that participants may wish to personally benefit from taking part in studies by receiving feedback on (personal) study results. In response to this, feedback has been provided to participants in a variety of ways. First, throughout the studies, participants could also see their own symptom data in the app (**Fig. 5**). In doing so, participants were able to constantly see the benefits of ongoing data completion in enabling them to track their own condition, to identify triggers of symptom flares or decline in health, and to improve communication with friends, family, and health care professionals[17]:

Making the observations for this study has made me aware of how much better I feel if I spend a reasonable amount of time out of doors, and moderately active.
—Cloudy with a Chance of Pain participant

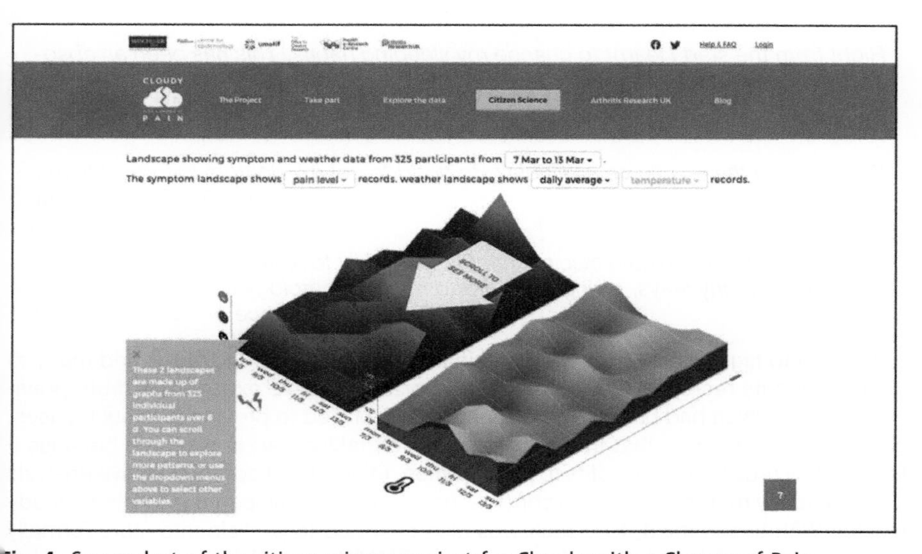
CLOUDY
PAIN
The Project
Take part
Explore the data
Citizen Science
Arthritis Research UK
Blog
Help & FAQ
Login
Landscape showing symptom and weather data from 325 participants from 7 Mar to 13 Mar
The symptom landscape shows pain level records. weather landscape shows daily average temperature records.
SCROLL TO SEE MORE

Fig. 4. Screenshot of the citizen science project for Cloudy with a Chance of Pain.

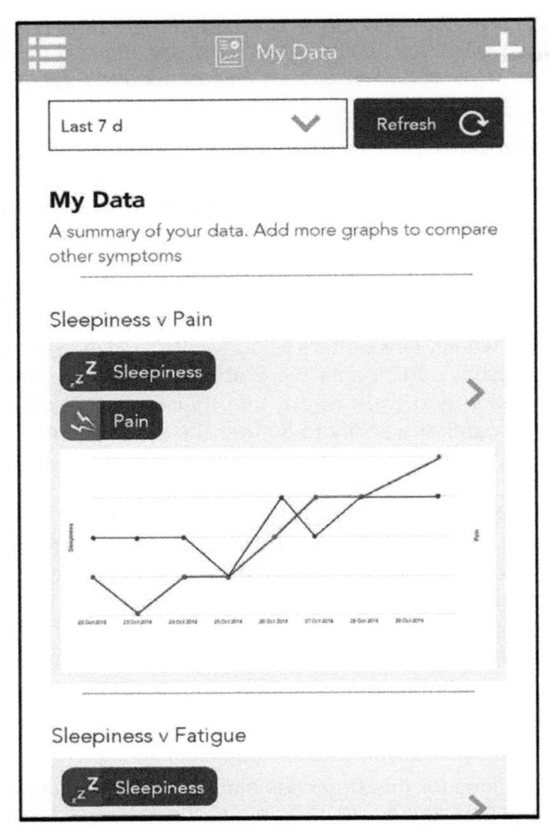

Fig. 5. Example participant feedback provided via the symptom tracking feature of the uMotif app.

> *Right from the start I learnt to change my sleeping habits. This has been an absolute life changer in coping with my pain.*
>
> *—QUASAR participant*

> *When would the results be available? Be good to get my doctors to look at them.*
>
> *—QUASAR participant*

> *I am finding the graph data fascinating. Plus it's great to have a chance to chart my illness in so many ways, giving new info to my rheumatology consultant.*
>
> *—Cloudy with a Chance of Pain participant*

It is vital to highlight that several participants in the PAG for QUASAR and many of the participants recruited to the study emphasized negative experiences from previous studies, which had promised feedback but had failed to provide it. In such cases, participants mentioned that they had been put off taking part in research because it felt like they received no benefits to participation. Mindful that comprehensive analysis can take many months, it is worth considering providing participants with interim study results. With this in mind, feedback was also provided to participants more formally within personalized end-of-study reports. In QUASAR, participants were provided with an end-of-study report that detailed their total hours of sleep each night for 1 week and their corresponding average pain, fatigue, and well-being scores. In Cloudy with a Chance of Pain, participants were invited to request a bespoke study postcard of their data, designed in collaboration with a creative researcher, which showed participants all of their symptoms reported throughout the 12-month study period (**Fig. 6** [*left*]) and the average of those symptoms over a monthly time period (see **Fig. 6** [*right*]).

Networking Effects and Community Building

The significance of creating a study community was highlighted within the Cloudy with a Chance of Pain study, in which various (optional) social media and support channels were also made available to participants to engage with the study team and other participants.

In the first instance, an online community (786 members and 107 posts) was established by the study team and hosted by HealthUnlocked, a UK patient support network. Within this community, participants (who may have been preexisting members of HealthUnlocked) could discuss their study experience and connect with other participants, to discuss their health more widely. There were no restrictions on what participants could discuss within the community, provided they followed HealthUnlocked's terms of use (https://healthunlocked.com/policies/terms).

Furthermore, participants were able to connect with the research team and other participants via the study team's presence on social media, including Twitter (@CloudyPain; 883 followers), Facebook (Cloudy with a Chance of Pain; 585 likes), and Instagram (@Cloudy_Pain; 49 followers). Finally, weekly newsletters and an online blog (https://www.cloudywithachanceofpain.com/blog) disseminated information about study progress and included guest articles from participants, charity partners, researchers, and funders. Importantly, by establishing the study community, it was possible to enable participants to feel empowered to share their experience.

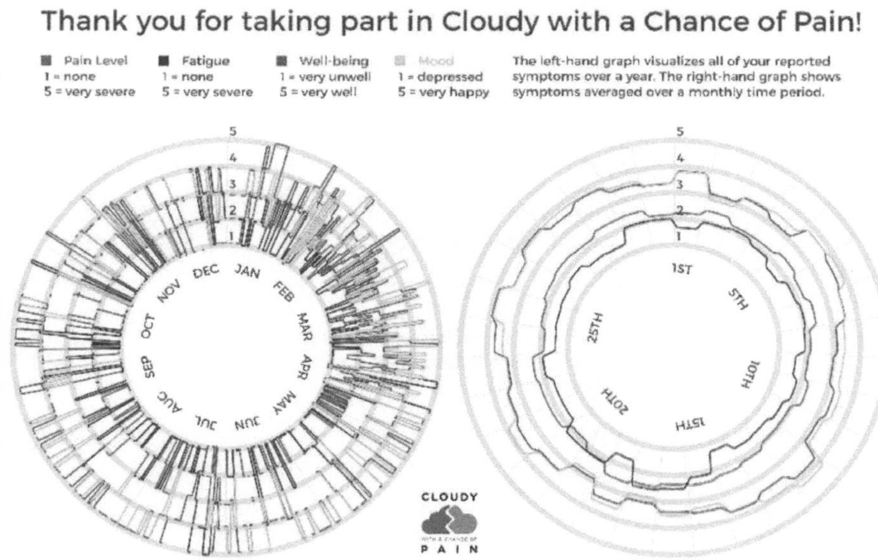

Fig. 6. Example participant feedback postcard provided in Cloudy with a Chance of Pain.

After the end of the study, all social media accounts remained live to promote dissemination of the final results of the study and any relevant interim findings. The community page on HealthUnlocked also remained live for participants to continue using at their discretion, but it was not actively monitored by the study team after the end of the study.

PERSONAL CONTACT AND ABILITY TO OBTAIN HELP

In addition to the support provided by study communities, personal, as opposed to virtual, contact was highlighted as an essential provision for mHealth studies. In particular, QUASAR PAG members believed that having personal contact was important to make participants feel valued and more likely to complete the data collection protocol. Specifically, PAG members recognized that many people may never have participated in mHealth studies before, and there was a need for ongoing reassurance and feeling that their participation is important. As a result, PAG members requested the development of processes to ensure participants had access to ongoing study support by phone or e-mail, courtesy calls, or check-ins during the study and ongoing feedback or study progress updates.

Although the experience of personal contact is preferred by participants, the decision to provide of courtesy calls or check-ins must be made in consideration of the study resources and the sample size to be recruited. For example, without substantial logistical support, it would have been impossible to provide courtesy calls to each of the 13,256 people recruited to Cloudy with a Chance of Pain. Due to staff capacity and study support, neither was it feasible for such calls to be made in the QUASAR study, but instead a decision was made to adopt the use of personalized motivational messages (ie, referring to the participant by name [**Fig. 7**]), which could be automatically generated and sent by a computer program but could offer support and opportunities

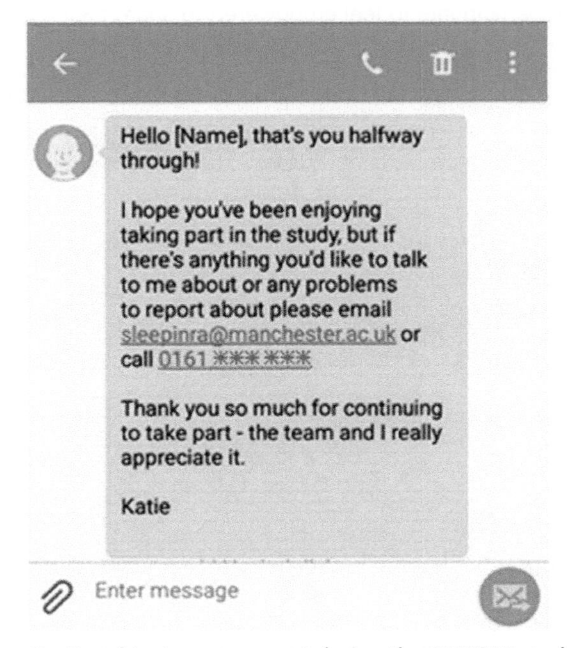

Fig. 7. Example motivational text message sent during the QUASAR study.

for participants to be telephoned by a member of the study team. Any contact requests were responded to within 24 hours, except in exceptional circumstances. In addition to e-mail support, participants were able to telephone both study teams at any stage in the study.

Participants were free to contact members of the study team to discuss any issues they wanted to, including concerns they had about the study or any technical difficulties they were experiencing. The only restriction was that no medical advice would be provided over the phone. Instances where participants contacted the study team tended to be to gain support for one-off issues, such as difficulty registering, reporting an inability to use the event marker on the sleep monitor, or to indicate their withdrawal from the study. A small group of people (n <20) made repeat contacts to the study team to discuss issues experienced throughout the study, including problems with data entry or study reminders, or to check that they were completing data correctly.

In addition to study-specific support, technical support was provided by the app providers, uMotif, via a designated help desk. A mutual sharing of relevant emails between the help desk and study team members ensured that any misdirected emails could still be responded to immediately (eg, requests for help with the sleep monitor sent to the uMotif help desk, instead of the QUASAR study team). As with the main study email account, help requests to uMotif were responded to within 24 hours to 48 hours, except in exceptional circumstances.

Investment in ongoing study support is integral to the success of future studies, because participants specifically identified the ability to obtain help as a factor for ongoing participation. In particular, within the QUASAR study, participants principally had 1 point of contact during the study, with the study coordinator responsible for all recruitment calls and participant contacts, and participants specifically highlighted this continuity of communication as a benefit of the study. Thea authors recommend such an approach be adopted, if feasible, within future mHealth studies.

SUMMARY

It is well recognized that mHealth technologies provide an exciting opportunity for researchers to obtain frequent and repeated measures for a range of self-report data and objective assessments and address hitherto unanswerable questions. Despite these benefits, mHealth studies are vulnerable to high attrition rates and it is essential that researchers actively consider strategies to maximize participant engagement. In 2 successful mHealth studies, the authors focused on factors associated with usability of technology, including functional ability of participants and consideration of participant workload and time commitment; push or motivating factors, such as the use of reminders and data monitoring; and the provision of personal contact and study support. Future studies should consider adopting and advancing these approaches at an early stage of study design to maximize engagement.

REFERENCES

1. Ofcom. Adults media use and attitudes report 2016. p. 23. Available at: https://www.ofcom.org.uk/__data/assets/pdf_file/0026/80828/2016-adults-media-use-and-attitudes.pdf.
2. Pew Research Centre. Mobile fact sheet. 2017. Available at: http://www.pewinternet.org/fact-sheet/mobile/. Accessed February 8, 2018.
3. Sama PR, Eapen ZJ, Weinfurt KP, et al. An evaluation of mobile health application tools. JMIR Mhealth Uhealth 2014;2:e19.

4. Honeyman M, Dunn P, McKenna H. A digital NHS? An introduction to the digital agenda and plans for implementation. London: King's Fund; 2016. p. 16.
5. Bot BM, Suver C, Neto EC, et al. The mPower study, Parkinson disease mobile data collected using ResearchKit. Sci Data 2016;3:160011.
6. Druce KL, Cordingley L, Short V, et al. Quality of life, sleep and rheumatoid arthritis (QUASAR): A protocol for a prospective UK mHealth study to investigate the relationship between sleep and quality of life in adults with rheumatoid arthritis. BMJ Open 2018;8:e018752.
7. Gliner V, Behar J, Yaniv Y. Novel method to efficiently create an mhealth app: implementation of a real-time electrocardiogram R peak detector. JMIR Mhealth Uhealth 2018;22:e118.
8. Losa-Iglesias ME, Becerro-de-Bengoa-Valleja R, Becerro-de-Bengoa-Losa KR. Reliability and concurrent validity of a peripheral pulse oximeter and health-app system for the quantification of heart rate in healthy adults. Health Informatics J 2014;22:151–9.
9. Eysenbach G. The law of attrition. J Med Internet Res 2005;7:e11.
10. Siegal J. Is Pokemon Go already dying?. 2016. Available at: https://bgr.com/2016/08/23/pokemon-go-daily-active-users/. Accessed October 9, 2018.
11. Perro J. Mobile apps: what's a good retention rate?. 2018. Available at: https://info.localytics.com/blog/mobile-apps-whats-a-good-retention-rate. Accessed October 30, 2018.
12. Crouthamel M, Quattrocchi E, Watts S, et al. Using a ResearchKit smartphone app to collect rheumatoid arthritis symptoms from real-world participants: feasibility study. JMIR Mhealth Uhealth 2018;6:e177.
13. McConnell MV, Shcherbine A, Pavlovic A, et al. Feasibility of obtaining measures of lifestyule from a smartphone app: the MyHeart counts cardiovascular health study. JAMA Cardiol 2017;2:67–76.
14. Silman AJ, Macfarlane GJ. Epidemiological Studies: a practical guide. 2nd edition. Cambridge (United Kingdom): Cambridge University Press; 2002.
15. Druce KL, McBeth J, van der Veer SN, et al. Recruitment and ongoing engagement in a UK smartphone study examining the association between weather and pain. JMIR Mhealth Uhealth 2017;5:e168.
16. Reade S, Spencer K, Sergeant J, et al. Engagement and subsequent attrition of daily data entry: Pilot smartphone study of weather, disease severity and physical activity in patients with rheumatoid arthritis. JMIR Mhealth Uhealth 2017;5:e37.
17. Dixon WG, Michaud K. Using technology to support clinical care and research in rheumatoid arthritis. Curr Opin Rheumatol 2018;30:276–81.
18. Mansournia MA, Etminan M, Kaufman JS. Handling time varying confounding in observational research. Bmj 2017;359:j4587.
19. Verhagen SJW, Hasmi L, Drukker M, et al. Use of the experience sampling method in the context of clinical trials. Evid Based Ment Health 2017;19:86–9.
20. Richardson JE, Reid MC. The Promises and Pitfalls of Leveraging Mobile Health Technology for Pain Care. Pain Medicine 2013;14(11):1621–6.
21. Dobkin BH, Dorsch A. The Promise of mHealth: Daily Activity Monitoring and Outcome Assessments by Wearable Sensors. Neurorehabilitation and Neural Repair 2011;25(9):788–98.
22. Slegers C, Zion D, Glass D, et al. Why do people participate in epidemiological research? J Bioeth Inq 2015;12:227–37.

Digital Interventions to Build a Patient Registry for Rheumatology Research

William Benjamin Nowell, PhD[a,*], David Curtis[a], Michelle Thai[b], Carole Wiedmeyer[a], Kelly Gavigan, MPH[a], Shilpa Venkatachalam, PhD[a], Seth Ginsberg[a], Jeffrey R. Curtis, MD, MS, MPH[c]

KEYWORDS

- Rheumatoid arthritis • Research recruitment • Patient-reported outcomes
- Patient-generated health data • Mobile technology • Symptom assessment
- Self-management • Data collection

KEY POINTS

- Digital interventions are effective for building a research registry community for patients with rheumatic and musculoskeletal disease.
- Different approaches and costs are associated with recruitment, engagement, and activation and each has variable effectiveness that can be measured.
- Registry recruitment and long-term engagement within a patient community, even one without preexisting research ties, is more effective than recruitment of "strangers" online.

BACKGROUND

Digital Tools Are Everywhere and Present Unprecedented Opportunities to Improve Health

Programs and devices using digital technology to prompt patients to take a health-related action or promote health behavior change are now widely used in medical care. They include mobile apps; Short Message Service (SMS) messages; wearable/ambient sensors; social media; and interactive Websites for diagnosis and treatment, disease prevention, and self-management. In addition to these resources for

Disclosures: No authors have any relevant conflicts of interest related to this work.

[a] Global Healthy Living Foundation, 515 North Midland Avenue, Upper Nyack, NY 10960, USA; [b] Media Cause, 147 Natoma Street, San Francisco, CA 94105, USA; [c] Division of Clinical Immunology & Rheumatology, University of Alabama at Birmingham, Faculty Office Tower, 510 20th Street South #834, Birmingham, AL 35294, USA
* Corresponding author. Global Healthy Living Foundation, 515 North Midland Avenue, Upper Nyack, NY 10960.
E-mail address: bnowell@ghlf.org

Rheum Dis Clin N Am 45 (2019) 173–186
https://doi.org/10.1016/j.rdc.2019.01.009 rheumatic.theclinics.com
0889-857X/19/

personal consumption, most if not all can be used to support and enrich research participation.[1,2]

At least in principle, the convenience and accessibility facilitated by digital technology should enable health care providers and researchers to collect traditional and novel types of health-related data more frequently than ever before in a more targeted and interesting way. An ethical responsibility to protect patients and human subjects accompanies these advances and has led to increased attention to privacy safeguards, secure data storage and transfer, and the importance of providing accurate and appropriate information to patients. Digitally delivered health-related interventions must support a desired behavior or interaction without distracting from or inhibiting other healthy behaviors. Efforts to develop robust digital health research technologies have necessarily focused on ethical oversight but lagged in fully realizing potential benefits to patient health and research.

Why Build a Research Community of People Living with Rheumatic and Musculoskeletal Disease?

Rheumatologic conditions, particularly those manifesting as inflammatory arthritis (eg, rheumatoid arthritis [RA], psoriatic arthritis, spondyloarthritis), can be debilitating, often causing pain, swelling, stiffness, and impediments in joint function along with structural joint damage.[3–7]

They typically strike younger people (median age 30s and 40s) in the prime of work and family productivity and are usually lifelong. There are genetic and environmental factors associated with the onset of these conditions, but there is no known cure. According to the Centers for Disease Control, arthritis is the leading cause of disability in the United States.[8,9]

Research has not answered many questions that patients with rheumatic and musculoskeletal diseases (RMDs) face or has failed to provide information in a format that patients can understand and use. Patients want to know: which treatments and behaviors are best for me given my individual values, characteristics, and circumstances? What are signs that my medication is not working? How does arthritis affect more than joints? How will my disease progress? What are the side effects of the available drugs to treat my RMD and which might be best for me?[10,11]

In recognition of the importance of filling evidence gaps in inflammatory arthritis-related and other RMD patient–centered research, CreakyJoints, a digital, patient-driven community, and rheumatology and informatics researchers at the University of Alabama at Birmingham (UAB) collaborated to develop a patient registry for adult RMD research using a digital platform.[12] The purpose of this article is to describe general principles and specific implementations of those principles, which were formative in building the registry, and then to describe the effect of those actions on developing the nascent ArthritisPower registry.

METHODS

Development of the "ArthritisPower" registry initially was supported by an award from the Patient-Centered Outcomes Research Institute and, subsequently, by more than a dozen externally funded studies. Originally referred to as *AR*thritis *P*artnership *W*ith Comparative *E*ffectiveness *R*esearchers Patient-Powered Research Network (AR-PoWER PPRN), ArthritisPower is one of 20 such PPRN registries within the national Patient-Centered Clinical Research Network (PCORnet), a US comparative effectiveness research network that spans multiple health conditions.[13] Developing the ArthritisPower registry consisted of 3 overlapping objectives: (1) to build a multipurpose digital platform ("app") for adult participants living with one or more RMDs to provide data, track their disease, and receive useful information; (2) to recruit, consent, and enroll participants into the registry; and (3) to activate participants' engagement with the registry app for research and related activities. The Institutional Review Boards of UAB and Schulman/Advarra provided oversight for protection of human subjects.

BUILDING A DIGITAL PLATFORM ("APP") FOR DATA COLLECTION AND PATIENT ENGAGEMENT

App Design Principles and Functionality

CreakyJoints and UAB researchers worked with both university-based (ie, UAB) and commercially employed software developers to construct a mobile application ("app") for iPhone and Android smartphones and a functionally equivalent Website at www.ArthritisPower.org. The technology serves multiple goals including obtaining consent, securely capturing patient data (eg, directly from patients via the phone or via electronic data imports and linkages [eg, with laboratory providers, electronic health record (EHR) system vendors, health plan claims data]), enabling patients to track their disease and its treatments, and engaging patients in research and education. The app was beta-tested early in 2015 with a small group of patient users and version 1.0 deployed for broader testing via a fully functional "soft launch" in March 2015. Consistent with principles of user-centered design,[14] the authors expected that they would have a minimally viable product that could be iterated on and improved with patient feedback.

During May to June 2015, usability testing was conducted to examine first-time users' experience with the app in order to (1) prioritize software enhancements for ArthritisPower, (2) identify barriers to registration and use, and (3) determine which version 1.0 components were most important to patients. An initial sampling frame of CreakyJoints members with RA or other inflammatory arthritis was selected who were representative across race/ethnicity (among white, African-American, Asian, and Latino members) and had not yet enrolled in ArthritisPower. Candidates for usability testing were invited via email that included a weblink to a brief screening tool and an interview scheduling survey. Usability testing interviews lasting 60 to 90 minutes were conducted via phone/Webex platform by 2 moderators (one research coordinator and one ArthritisPower Patient Governor[12]) following a guide. Interviewers led users in a "think aloud" protocol to elicit feedback while using the web-based version of ArthritisPower on a computer or tablet; they prompted users with questions as needed to generate additional comments. Email correspondence was completed with the participants before and after to confirm participation and to follow-up for patient incentive ($25 each for their participation). Each interview was recorded (audio and video of screen) using GoToMeeting. Moderators also took notes during each interview and added information to their notes when reviewing the recordings. Content of the typed notes was analyzed to identify themes for recommendations. Synthesized recommendations were shared with the research team and software development team. Recommendations were classified by the larger team as being high-, medium-, or low-level priority based on the following criteria: (1) the number of people who made the comment/suggestion (generalizability), (2) evaluation of whether the feedback represented new feature development vs improvement of existing features, with the latter prioritized, (3) potential impact on improving effectiveness of marketing and recruitment, (4) potential impact on smoothing registration barriers, and (5) anticipated ease of implementation and resource requirements.

More than 2000 participants were recruited to the registry during the first 6 months to obtain user feedback on the deployed minimally viable product. A significant redesign of the app was then undertaken during the following 18 months to incorporate the synthesized and prioritized recommendations before releasing version 2.0 in April 2017 (**Fig. 1**). As clarified during this period, the design goals for the ArthritisPower software platform included 4 main pillars. Features responsive to each of these core pillars are described here.

Personal longitudinal health and medication tracking

The app was developed to enable active and passive data collection for both structured and unstructured data, including health tracking measures (eg, patient-reported outcomes [PROs]) and medications. ArthritisPower collects comprehensive data about patients enrolled in the network in a way that allows the app to be highly personalized to individual patients, consistent with the concept of "participatory design."[2] Each patient can select the aspect of their health they want to track longitudinally from a library of more than 80 electronic PRO measures (e-PROMs) from both computer adaptive testing (CAT) PROMIS instruments,[15] plus a variety of rheumatology-specific short-form instruments (eg, RAPID3, BASDAI, flare). Patients may also log symptom notes organized by date to provide context to their symptoms. To track status over time, patients can view results graphically and generate tailored reports that are exportable from the app.

The initial version of ArthritisPower (1.0) collected data only on a selected list of RMD medications. However, based on substantial user feedback (see later discussion), the medication tracking feature was reengineered to enable participants to track medications by selecting from a complete list of options based on the RxNorm ontology. Part of the Unified Medical Language System, RxNorm provides information on drug ingredients, generic and brand names, and relationships with other medications and therapeutic classes.[16] In addition to symptom and medication tracking, patients report demographic data during the initial registration and contribute patient preference or other data via customized surveys through integration with the SurveyMonkey application programming interface, a "communication pipeline" between 2 different

Home Screen with Notification

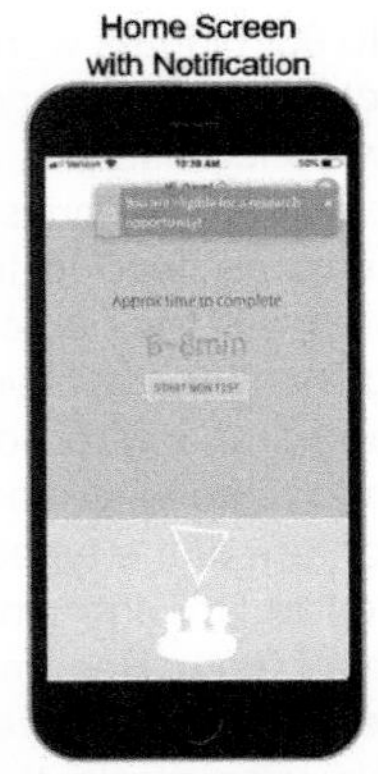

After login, participant is presented with home screen to:

- "Start New Test", the core health assessment feature
- View research notifications or announcements
- Access main navigation

Health Assessments

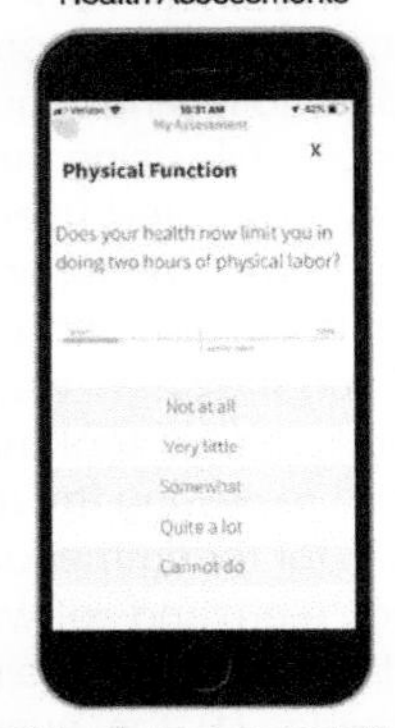

Participant is then presented with queue of health assessments (measures) based on active study cohort(s). Participant may select additional instruments for symptom tracking to include in their assessment queue, if they choose.

Health Picture Summary

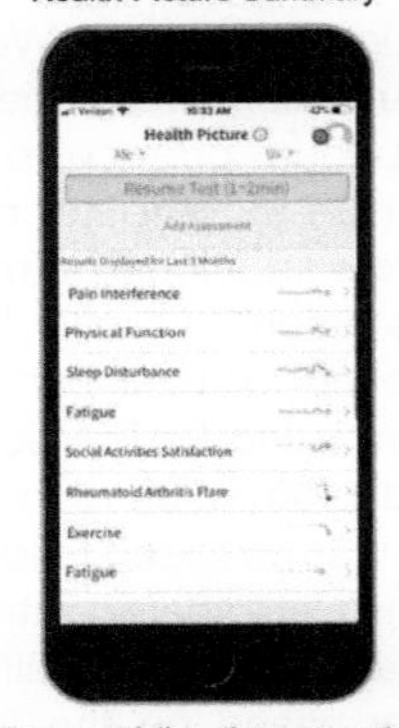

Upon completion of assessment queue, participant is presented with a summary of all individual health assessment scores (quick view of overall health and trends). Date range can be adjusted by participant. This view display shows results from the last 3 mo.

Fig. 1. ArthritisPower app: core functionality.

software applications, embedded within the app. The ArthritisPower consent form includes an electronic medical record release and HIPAA authorization to allow patients' data to be imported into the ArthritisPower app for use by patients and shared with the registry. This approach facilitates linkages to EHR data, laboratory results, and claims data for clinical and research purposes. For example, an agreement was established with Crescendo Bioscience to import RA patients' VectraDA scores (a validated biomarker-based test that tracks RA disease activity)[3] and make these data available for patient viewing in app and for research purposes.

Collectively, these features enabled patients to record and view a comprehensive picture of their disease activity outside of physician visits and allow extensive PRO data capture, easy assessment of participants' opinions, and participant choice in measure and frequency of administration from a library of instruments.

Health care decision-making

The app was also designed to optimize patient-provider engagement through longitudinal viewing and sharing of health reports. The "Health Picture" function allows participants to view their responses to PRO measures over time to gauge how their symptoms responded to changes in treatment or other factors (eg, lifestyle changes). Participants can customize reports to include medications as well as vary the type and frequency of their preferred PRO measures, with the ability to share this information (eg, in-app, paper, or email) with their doctor or others (eg, caregivers). This feature enables them to use their own data in discussions with their health care team. The authors are currently conducting a funded pilot that links their data with a large EHR vendor that supports more than 500 community rheumatologists. This enables the data to be most effectively used at the point of care with seamless integration with the EHR and consideration of impact on the workflow of busy clinical practices to maximize the utility of the data for health care decision-making.

Research opportunities

Although the registry infrastructure provides a robust platform with which to conduct research, its potential is maximized through ancillary studies nested within the registry context. These can be proposed by any researcher and undergo review by both the Patient Governor Group and members of the ArthritisPower Research Advisory Board for patient centeredness, scientific rigor, and public health impact. A formal process has been put in place to propose, review, refine, and execute ancillary studies, which takes advantage of the infrastructure created that maximizes interactions with researchers and patient and patient advocate stakeholders.

At the time of login, participants are greeted with the latest opportunities to engage in ancillary study projects, tailored to patient's health condition, geography, PRO data, medication use, and other health-related features. This customization allows such opportunities to be offered in a highly tailored fashion based on individuals' expected eligibility and is efficient from a participant burden perspective. For example, women younger than 40 years with RA treated with certain RA medications might be invited to participate in a pregnancy and family planning–related ancillary study that (based on its eligibility criteria) would not be offered to other participants and therefore not waste their time sifting through irrelevant invitations. Additional projects are being conducted that consume biosensor and wearable device data to make it available within the app and use it alongside other research data collected by the app or at clinical visits.

Patient engagement, community integration, and education

Among notable findings from preliminary discussions with CreakyJoints patients, it was found that many patients had not previously had the opportunity to discuss their condition with others. Thus, community integration became a fundamental pillar to ensure that CreakyJoints blogger content and ongoing CreakyJoints Twitter discussions on diverse topics affecting our patient community was available through a "tabbed" menu on the app's opening screen. In addition, the authors worked with a national digital education provider to provide state-of-the-art and timely education to our members. The ArthritisPower app included a "Send Feedback" option to inform changes affecting the functionality and usability of the app to better align the app with user-participant preferences. User suggestions guided development as prioritized by feedback from the advisory boards of researchers and patients (the ArthritisPower Research Advisory Board and Patient Governor Group), the broader CreakyJoints patient community, and the needs and requirements of the PCORnet infrastructure. These stakeholders' views were solicited so as to better align the app with user/participant preferences, ensure more robust and efficient data collection mechanisms that considered participant burden, and fulfill the intended goals of the registry. The app design thus follows the principles of user-centered/participatory design with our patient community.[14,17] Therefore, even with secure methods in place to protect data privacy, participation in ArthritisPower is a social experience. CreakyJoints social media channels and blogs can be viewed in app, seamlessly.

Data Storage and Privacy

Rather than being stored on a patient's smartphone, ArthritisPower data are stored in secure servers located within the HIPAA-compliant Amazon Web Services' data centers. A mirror of the identifiable ArthritisPower data is housed in a protected, secure fashion at the University of Alabama at Birmingham and protected within the same secure environment as other university health system data. This server infrastructure has full 24-hour monitoring, disaster recovery, and redundancy in case of unexpected issues. Privacy and confidentiality provisions are guided by ArthritisPower's data use agreements and conform to a "minimum necessary requirement," a key protection of the HIPAA Privacy Rule.[18] Importantly, data can remain identifiable or (more commonly) can be partially or fully deidentified for analysis by the principal investigators of ancillary studies conducted within the registry.

RECRUITING, CONSENTING, ENGAGING, AND ACTIVATING PARTICIPANTS FOR RESEARCH

An online enrollment process and informed consent process including digital capture of the participant's signature were created to facilitate ArthritisPower registration. The consent form is presented to potential participants on a single webpage requiring potential participants to scroll to read the full document. A copy of the signed consent was stored in Portable Document Format and available for consented individuals to reference in the "Profile" section of the app on logging in, and therefore, no paper forms are required.

Two different general approaches were used for registry recruitment from within, and outside, the CreakyJoints patient community. The approach within the CreakyJoints patient community entailed growing and nurturing members of the CreakyJoints online arthritis patient community (the primary ArthritisPower sampling frame) over time before inviting them to join the research registry. Recruitment outside of the CreakyJoints community entailed a direct ask of members of the public and online "strangers" (ie, not known to CreakyJoints) to join ArthritisPower. The relative effectiveness of each approach at driving ArthritisPower registration was assessed and is described later.

Recruitment from Within the CreakyJoints Patient Community

Within patient community recruitment involved a 3-step process of (1) growing the size of the CreakyJoints patient community eligible and available for registry recruitment; (2) nurturing a closer relationship with these individuals by providing helpful information and resources to them and highlighting important evidence gaps, with the anticipated effect to foster greater interest in research participation; and (3) inviting CreakyJoints community members to join ArthritisPower.

To grow CreakyJoints membership, search engine optimization (SEO), Google Search Ads, Facebook ads, and other social media were deployed to reach people interested in RMD-related content and prompt them to be part of the CreakyJoints community where joining requires only that one share a valid email address. The authors hypothesized that SEO tactics would work well to grow CreakyJoints because 80% of Internet users, or about 93 million Americans, have searched for a health-related topic online.[19] Using tools such as Google Keyword Planner and Google Trends, the authors created content for topics that showed high search volume; among the conditions relevant to CreakyJoints, RA, gout, and AS had averages of 301,000, 450,000, and 135,000 searches per month, respectively. Then when a person used Google to search for advice on living with RA, a relevant email capture (via a pop-up or slider) encourages her to subscribe to CreakyJoints when she views the relevant links returned by Google. In addition to SEO efforts, Google Search Ads were used to target people based on what they are searching for. Google gives a $10,000 per month grant to 501(c)3 not-for-profit organizations such as GHLF/CreakyJoints, and the ads drive people to email-gated content (ie, content that requires subscribing to CreakyJoints with an email address to access).

Once new CreakyJoints members were subscribed to the online community, subscribers' affinity with CreakyJoints was nurtured with relevant, valuable information. CreakyJoints members received a welcome email and were then engaged over weeks and months via email series and content tailored to their interests. Most automated email series were 3 to 9 emails long and included the following: Day 1-Thank you for subscribing; Day 3-Tips on living with (health condition); Day 7-Important insurance issues you may encounter in your patient journey; and Day 14-Contributing to research. CreakyJoints members received other regular email content including a periodic newsletter ("CreakyJoints News") with content such as announcements of new drugs approved by the Food and Drug Administration, advice on living with RA or other RMDs, issues patients may encounter with prior authorization challenges for medications, and personal accounts about coping with chronic conditions by patient writers.

During these email interactions, CreakyJoints members were provided with information about ArthritisPower and encouraged to learn more. Seasonal events and key milestones were leveraged to ask members of the patient community to join ArthritisPower. For example, CreakyJoints members received an email during Arthritis Awareness Month encouraging them to do more than just raise awareness and to join ArthritisPower; an email in December/January nudged them to "Track changes in your pain this winter" using ArthritisPower; and periodic emails highlighted registry milestones such as the fact that "x" number of their patient-peers had joined ArthritisPower. Behavioral economic principles (eg, social norms) guided messaging to members.[20]

Recruitment Outside the Existing Patient Community

Several tactics were used for recruiting beyond the CreakyJoints patient community, an approach where individuals are directly invited to join ArthritisPower without a prior relationship with CreakyJoints. First, ArthritisPower ads on Facebook were posted, monitored, and adjusted in a dynamic process of "segmenting and optimizing." The authors started by segmenting the potential patient-participant audience to understand which ads would resonate with each segment. Cost per acquisition is a term used in digital marketing to refer to the investment required to attract a new customer. A similar concept is used to continuously assess cost per new participant registration to inform decisions about starting, stopping, adjusting, and creating new ads.

Second, ads were placed in niche publications (print and online). As an example, GHLF paid for placements with Pain-Free Living (PFL), a consumer magazine with a readership of 2 million individuals, of which 81% report having osteoarthritis and 25% RA. ArthritisPower ads and "advertorials" appeared in PFL magazine, banner ads scrolled on their Website, and ArthritisPower recruitment emails were sent to their contact list. Each of these ads, posts, or messages included a short, custom link to enable attribution of registrations back to PFL.

Third, organizational partners sent emails to their eligible patient members or posted information about ArthritisPower in organizational newsletters. Fourth, public relations initiatives, such as posting press releases on the wire and earning feature news stories, were leveraged to drive "strangers" to the ArthritisPower homepage where they saw more information about the registry and were prompted to sign up.

Finally, follow-up emails were sent to those individuals who started but did not complete registration, which first requires that potential participants submit an email address, including to those who had entered an email address on any of the customized ArthritisPower landing pages. A follow-up email was sent to everyone who had "abandoned registration" to tell them more about ArthritisPower and encourage them to return and complete registration.

Engaging with and Activating Participants

The next challenge was urging participants to provide their personal and PRO data over time to support generation of useful research. To do this, the registry sought to enhance patient engagement and activation by providing value to patients in several ways. Similar to recruitment, the authors hypothesized that engaging participants over time with communications and offering resources that they found valuable would increase the likelihood that they would respond to the more direct and immediate activation prompts.

ArthritisPower participants can go months without being invited to participate in a new ancillary study. To prompt them to update their medication and PRO data, monthly email reminders are sent. To keep them generally engaged in registry-related activities even in the absence of a particular study, monthly webinars on clinical and research-related topics are conducted (eg, how to talk to your doctor, pregnancy considerations relevant for patients with RMD) and biannual newsletters, community questions, and a periodic, individualized summary of their participation are sent. To assess level of participant engagement and activation, the authors track email open and click rates and frequencies and recency of in-app data contribution.

RESULTS

As of January 2019, more than 17,500 users had signed consent and joined the ArthritisPower research registry via mobile or digitally equivalent Website. Most of the growth followed release of version 2.0 of the ArthritisPower app in April 2017 and increased investment in implementing digital recruitment strategies such as Facebook and email campaigns (**Fig. 2**). The ArthritisPower participant population grew from

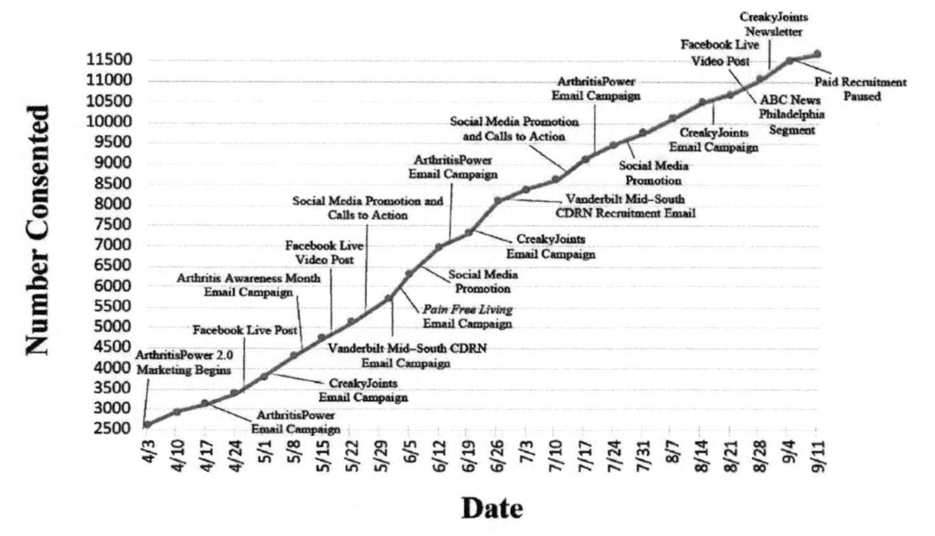

Fig. 2. Registry growth during 23-week period after launch of ArthritisPower (app 2.0).

2641 to 11,692 between April 4, 2017 and September 11, 2017. Although participation in the general registry is accessible to the entire population of greater than 17,500 patients, more than a dozen nested (ancillary) studies have been launched with specific subpopulations of ArthritisPower participants, with sample sizes ranging from 110 to more than 1000 participants.

For the usability testing to guide the app redesign process from 2016 to early 2017, the authors selected a sampling frame of CreakyJoints members with complete CreakyJoints registration information who were representative across race/ethnicity and were not yet enrolled as ArthritisPower participants. After removing the 10.7% of individuals who opted out of receiving emails directly from CreakyJoints and filtering and selection based on our screening criteria (eg, smartphone ownership), usability testing was conducted with a dozen patients. Participants from usability testing liked that the ArthritisPower app allowed them to contribute to research in an innovative way, linked with CreakyJoints, included a useful symptom tracking feature, and the fact that the registration site was uncluttered and generally easy to use. One participant said, "It gives us a way to help with the research that we all hope will make us well someday."

Five overall suggested improvements surfaced. First, participants recommended that the authors update the registration/consent process to clarify what is expected from registry participants and to emphasize that providing a Social Security number (SSN) is optional. Second, they were encouraged to add more instructional and explanatory text so users would know how to use the app: intro text on the dashboard to give an overview of app functionality, instructions in the Track feature (such as explaining frequency of PRO data capture and how to vary it), and an explanation of Research Opportunities. Third, the authors were recommended to improve their Results descriptions including better visualization of the Health Picture display. Fourth, they were encouraged to add more Opportunities for research activities to get patients accustomed to checking that section regularly. Fifth, and heard most frequently, they were asked to allow participants to select from and track a more comprehensive list of treatment options beyond only rheumatology medications and to simplify medication entry (especially dose).

These suggestions, along with other improvements identified from the "Send Feedback" option of the ArthritisPower app, which had garnered more than 576 comments by December 2017, were used to identify problems and inform software upgrades. Participants provided direct feedback to the research and development staff regarding the app and their experience using the "Send Feedback" function. The ArthritisPower team examined these feedback submissions and categorized them to identify common issues. These included issues with the registration process, app stability, navigation and ease of use, understanding of health assessments (eg, PRO measures), and medication entry.

In response to the request of patients expressing the desire to list all their active and past medications and not only their rheumatologic treatments, the medication entry functionality was completely reengineered. In the updated version 2.0, participants were newly able to select from a complete list of pharmaceutical and complementary medicine options using the RxNorm ontology. The level of detail in RxNorm that was presented to patients was piloted with patients to make final decisions because the authors observed that with too many choices, patients became unable to differentiate among closely named formulations of the same drug and often resorted to entering free text rather than selecting from the structured pick list. The medication tracking function also prompts patients to report their reasons for stopping or changing medications in broad categories (eg, inadequate efficacy, safety, tolerability, cost/administrative, and other). Additional recommendations not yet fully realized but which were in queue to implement were not just to capture information about medication frequency, but to enable an in-app reminder system service for RMD treatments taken at periodic intervals (eg, once weekly, once monthly).

Designing a User-Friendly Registration and Consent Process

To respond to patient suggestions to clarify the registration process and to address the concerns of the research team that many participants were simply clicking "Next" to continue registration without fully grasping what ArthritisPower enrollment entailed, the registration process was redesigned. Before advancing to the consent form, patients are able to read and click through a series of Overview pages describing the registry and what participation entails. The final of these webpages/screens includes 5 statements with check boxes to confirm that individuals have a basic understanding of the ArthritisPower registry before advancing to read and sign the full informed consent document (**Fig. 3**). In the consent and later when the participant completes registration fields with their personal information, it is made clear that providing SSN is optional and that omitting this information would not affect their status in the registry.

The registration redesign involved bringing important details to the forefront such as addressing common user concerns that surfaced from participant (or potential participant) feedback during registration (ie, security, privacy, and identity of GHLF and ArthritisPower team members) and following user experience best practices (eg, optimal font size, clean design). The redesigned registration process launched in early 2017 was described as "less intimidating" and "more friendly" by ArthritisPower participants.

Recruitment

The app and registration redesign, along with a variety of other recruitment efforts, allowed registration to grow from 0.43% of recruitment email recipients in 2016 to

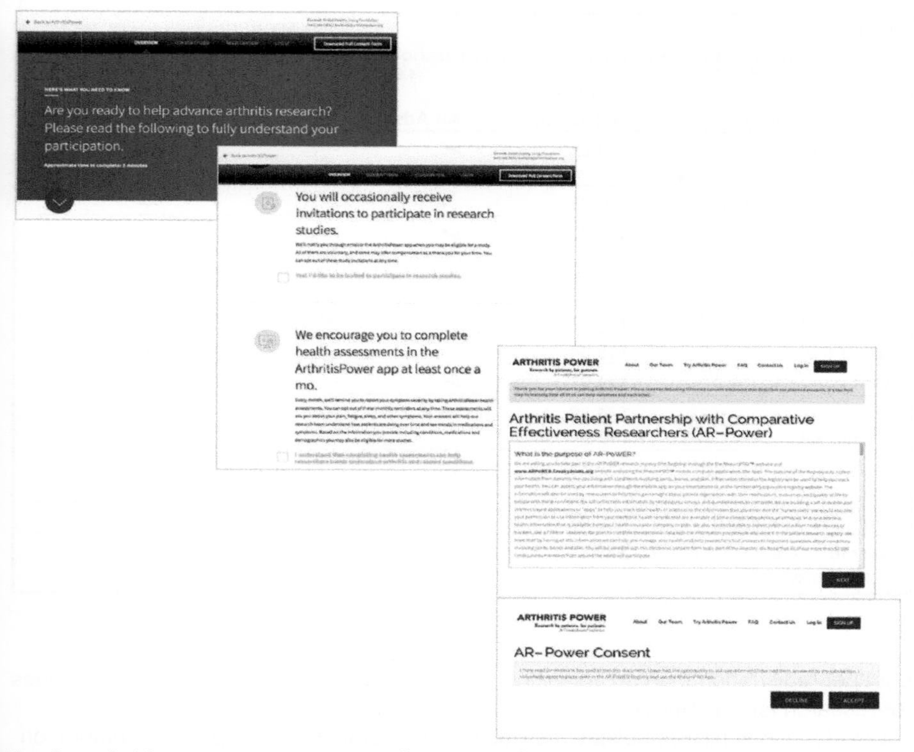

Fig. 3. ArthritisPower registration: confirmation of understanding before proceeding to consent.

8.21% in 2017. Overall, recruitment within the CreakyJoints patient community was nearly twice as effective as recruitment beyond the patient community. One-fifth (19.46%) of people who were referred to ArthritisPower by a CreakyJoints email ended up registering compared with less than one-eighth (11.53%) of people registered who joined ArthritisPower directly from a Facebook ad. The cost is comparatively low to subscribe new CreakyJoints members. One such campaign had a $2.39 cost per CreakyJoints subscriber from a Facebook ad campaign promoting the "Patient Guidelines Download (February 2018)." Recruiting to the registry in tandem with ads promoting a resource for useful information (ie, patient guidelines) was frequently used to attract potential participants beyond the existing patient community. Google Search Ads were also used to target people based on what they are searching for. The ads drive people to email-gated content, which requires subscribing to CreakyJoints to access. Ads result in roughly half of new CreakyJoints subscriptions annually; for example, 52% of new CreakyJoints subscribers came from our Google Search Ads during January 1 to December 31, 2018.

From "segmenting and optimizing," where cost per new participant registration by audience type was evaluated, the authors calculated their return on investment in digital marketing tactics. The average cost per registration (CPR) for Facebook ads was $34, with the lowest CPR at $10 for white women with RA and highest at $88 for men with gout (**Table 1**). Among women with RA aged 55 years and older, the authors found that an ArthritisPower Facebook ad displaying a sample question drove a lower

Table 1
Cost per registration (CPR) for ArthritisPower Facebook ads by audience (April 2018)

Target Audience	Cost Per Registration	All Ads	Flare "Sample Question" Ad	"Clues for Research" Ad
White women age 35+, RA	$10.09	✓	—	—
Women age 55+, RA	$10.33	—	✓	—
Men and women age 35+, PsA	$10.82	✓	—	—
Women age 55+, RA	$11.68	—	—	✓
Women age 35–54, RA	$12.51	—	✓	—
Women age 35–54, RA	$15.64	—	—	✓
Men age 35+, RA	$21.61	✓	—	—
Women of color age 55+, RA	$34.29	✓	—	—
Men and women age 35+, AS	$39.65	✓	—	—
Men age 35+, gout	$88.46	✓	—	—
Average CPR, all audiences	*$34.15*	✓	—	—

cost per registration than an ad asking about turning a patient's symptoms into clues for research (see **Table 1**).

CPR for ads in niche publications was higher overall. For example, the authors' online and print campaign with PFL had a CPR of $70.51 for the online tactics alone.

The authors also evaluated the return on following up via email with potential ArthritisPower participants who had abandoned their registration before completing it. One hundred thirty-two registrations came from the first abandoned follow-up email campaign sent between January 1 and Sept 30, 2018, plus another 39 registrations from the second abandoned email. A total of 171 of all 5845 registrations during the period meant the "abandoned registration email" approach drove 3% of total registrations, at minimal incremental cost.

Engagement/Activation for Data Collection

The authors found that the average overall open rate for all regular emails that go out to ArthritisPower participants list is approximately 16%. They therefore benchmark all ArthritisPower engagement and activation email messages against this open rate. If the content and format of an email yields the same or higher open rate after testing, it becomes part of ongoing ArthritisPower email communications, and if the open rate is lower, they stop.

Participants were also encouraged to permit collection of passive data via the smartphone app by providing additional rationale on how that data type serves a credible research purpose. For example, geolocation data provide additional information that enables comparisons of participants by geographic region, connects them to local patients and resources in their area, and provides correlation of weather and symptom data. Most participants have opted in to provide geolocation data. As of November 2018, of the 10,323 users who had encountered the location prompt that was sent to their smartphone device, 86.8% agreed to provide this data.

SUMMARY

Digital interventions are effective for building a research registry community for patients with RMD. Different approaches and costs are associated with recruitment, engagement, and activation and each have variable effectiveness that can be measured. In summary, (1) long-term engagement connected to a patient community (without preexisting research ties) and nurturing a relationship with them is more effective than recruitment of "strangers" online; (2) different target populations have different costs associated with their recruitment; coupling invitations to join the registry with a broad panoply of engaging content and opportunities seems to have the best yield; and (3) regular, tailored touchpoints with participants help build community and make it more likely they respond to an "ask" or call to action to join a registry, provide data, or participate in a study. Given these successes, the many participants and team members who support ArthritisPower are enthusiastic to continue to evolve it as a resource for patients and their clinicians to track health for clinical care, assist in improving quality, and answer high-impact clinical rheumatology research questions that matter to patients, clinicians, and other key stakeholders.

ACKNOWLEDGMENTS

This work was supported through a (Patient-Centered Outcomes Research Institute (PCORI), Washington, DC, USA) award (PPRN-1306-04811). All statements in this article, including its findings and conclusions, are solely those of the authors and do not necessarily represent the views of PCORI, its Board of Governors or Methodology Committee. The authors would like to thank CreakyJoints and ArthritisPower participants, and ArthritisPower Patient Governors, for their contribution to this project.

REFERENCES

1. Michie S, Yardley L, West R, et al. Developing and evaluating digital interventions to promote behavior change in health and health care: recommendations resulting from an international workshop. J Med Internet Res 2017;19(6):e232.
2. Alkhaldi G, Hamilton FL, Lau R, et al. The effectiveness of technology-based strategies to promote engagement with digital interventions: a systematic review protocol. J Med Internet Res 2015;17(5):e47.
3. Singh JA, Saag KG, Bridges SL, et al. 2015 American College of Rheumatology guideline for the treatment of rheumatoid arthritis. Arthritis Rheumatol 2016;68(1): 1–26.
4. Englund M, Joud A, Geborek P, et al. Prevalence and incidence of rheumatoid arthritis in southern Sweden 2008 and their relation to prescribed biologics. Rheumatology (Oxford) 2010;49(8):1563–9.
5. Myasoedova E, Davis JM, Crowson CS, et al. Epidemiology of rheumatoid arthritis: rheumatoid arthritis and mortality. Curr Rheumatol Rep 2010;12(5):379–85.
6. Neovius M, Simard JF, Askling J, ARTIS study group. Nationwide prevalence of rheumatoid arthritis and penetration of disease-modifying drugs in Sweden. Ann Rheum Dis 2011;70(4):624–9.
7. Symmons D, Turner G, Webb R, et al. The prevalence of rheumatoid arthritis in the United Kingdom: new estimates for a new century. Rheumatology (Oxford) 2002;41(7):793–800.

8. Gossec L, Dougados M, Goupille P, et al. Prognostic factors for remission in early rheumatoid arthritis: a multiparameter prospective study. Ann Rheum Dis 2004; 63(6):675–80.
9. CDC. Addressing the Nation's Most Common Cause of Disability At A Glance 2015. Centers for Disease Control and Prevention, Chronic Disease Prevention and Health Promotion: At A Glance Fact Sheets-Arthritis [Web page]. 2015. Available at: https://www.cdc.gov/chronicdisease/resources/publications/aag/pdf/2015/athritis-aag-508.pdf. Accessed May 18, 2016.
10. Nowell WB, Ginsberg S, Higginbotham P, et al. FRI0603 Patients' prioritization of patient-centered education and research topics in rheumatic disease. Ann Rheum Dis 2016;75(Suppl 2):660–1.
11. Fraenkel L, Miller AS, Clayton K, et al. When patients write the guidelines: patient panel recommendations for the treatment of rheumatoid arthritis. Arthritis Care Res 2016;68(1):26–35.
12. Nowell WB, Curtis JR, Crow-Hercher R. Patient governance in a patient-powered research network for adult rheumatologic conditions. Med Care 2018;56(Suppl 10 Suppl 1):S16–21.
13. Fleurence RL, Beal AC, Sheridan SE, et al. Patient-powered research networks aim to improve patient care and health research. Health Aff (Millwood) 2014; 33(7):1212–9.
14. Muller MJ. Participatory design: the third space in HCI. In: Jacko JA, Sears A, editors. Human-computer interaction: development process. Boca Raton (FL): CRC Press; 2009. p. 166–81.
15. Witter JP. Introduction: PROMIS a first look across diseases. J Clin Epidemiol 2016;73:87–8.
16. NIH: US National Library of Medicine. Unified Medical Language System (UMLS), RxNorm [Web page]. Available at: https://www.nlm.nih.gov/research/umls/rxnorm/overview.html. Accessed March 5, 2019.
17. Erwin K, Krishnan JA. Using design methods to provide the care that people want and need. J Comp Eff Res 2016;5(1):13–5.
18. Available at: http://www.hhs.gov/ocr/privacy/hipaa/understanding/coveredentities/minimumnecessary.html. Accessed April 1, 2015.
19. Fox S, Duggan M. Health Online 2013. Washington, DC: Pew Research Center; 2013. Available at: http://www.pewinternet.org/2013/01/15/health-online-2013/.
20. Dholakia UM, Bagozzi RP, Pearo LK. A social influence model of consumer participation in network- and small-group-based virtual communities. International Journal of Research in Marketing 2004;21(3):241–63.

Patient Self-Management and Tracking

A European Experience

Piet L.C.M. van Riel, MD, PhD[a,b,*], Rixt M. Zuidema, MSc[a], Carine Vogel, RN[a], Sanne A.A. Rongen-van Dartel, PhD[a,b]

KEYWORDS

- Self-management • Inflammatory rheumatic diseases • Digital tool • PROMs
- Education • Patients' experiences • Personalized health care

KEY POINTS

- There is a shift from a paternalistic model of health care toward more personalized health care in which disease management is conducted by the patient together with his or her health professional.
- Self-management by patients can be performed in various levels including being prepared for an outpatient clinic visit with a list of current medications and suggesting to the health care professional to lower the dosage of a prescribed medication.
- Remote control by self-monitoring might give important information about the disease course between outpatient clinic visits. Outpatient visits can be minimized when patients monitor their disease activity themselves using a digital tool like Reumanet.
- For self-management, it is important to have an easy to understand electronic health record with a well-organized dashboard informing both the patient as well as the health professional about the status of the different domains.
- At the outpatient clinic, the doctor should discuss the results of the self-management and self-monitoring with the patient.

INTRODUCTION

More than 2500 years ago, the ancient Greeks like Hippocrates realized that maintaining good health and managing diseases depended on the natural causes and lifestyle issues like diet and exercise as well as on the environment.[1] Already at that time, a lot of attention was being given to educate the population, to teach them that diseases

All authors declare to have no conflict of interest. No funding was obtained for this article.
[a] Department of Rheumatology, Bernhoven, Uden, the Netherlands; [b] Radboud University Medical Center, Radboud Institute for Health Sciences, Scientific Institute for Quality of Healthcare (IQ Healthcare), Nijmegen, the Netherlands
* Corresponding author. Radboud University Medical Center, Radboud Institute for Health Sciences, IQ healthcare, Nijmegen, the Netherlands.
E-mail address: piet.vanriel@radboudumc.nl

Rheum Dis Clin N Am 45 (2019) 187–195
https://doi.org/10.1016/j.rdc.2019.01.008 rheumatic.theclinics.com
0889-857X/19/

are influenced by emotional factors, and that human behavior has a strong influence on the course of diseases. Special educators went to villages to increase the so-called self-sufficiency of the population, which we now would call patient self-management. In the twentieth century, due to the 1948 World Health Organization definition of health, "health is a state of *complete* physical, mental and social well-being and not merely the absence of disease or infirmity," the focus was to find medical solutions to cure each disease. This fitted in the paternalistic approach, which was the standard procedure for how medicine was practiced: the doctor is dominant and makes decisions for the patient.

In the past decade, we moved from this paternalistic approach to a shared decision model in which the patient together with the health care professional make the decisions. This fits more in the new definition for positive health, which "is the ability to *adapt* and to *self-manage*, in the face of social, physical and emotional challenges."[2] In the same period, it has been shown that lifestyle factors do influence the development of the disease, the course, and the response to treatments.[3–7] All these factors have caused more attention to be given to the role of the patient in the management of the disease. An important component of self-management is called self-monitoring, a patient undertakes self-measurement of, for instance, vital signs like weight and blood pressure or symptoms like pain, fatigue, and disease activity by Patient Reported Outcome Measures (PROM).[8,9]

The degree of self-management can vary per patient and depends for instance also on the situation the patient is facing. In an acute, life-threatening situation like a myocardial infarction, the degree of self-management of a patient at the emergency department will be minimal, whereas for patients with a chronic disease, the degree of self-management might vary between attending the outpatient clinic prepared with a list of their current medication usage to even suggesting to the health care professional to lower the dosage of a prescribed medication because their disease activity is low. Several studies have shown that patients with a chronic disease who practice self-monitoring do have a better outcome of their disease.[10] This, together with an improved cost-effectiveness of this approach, is the reason that self-management should be stimulated in patients with chronic diseases. Different studies, however, have shown that the percentage of patients with inflammatory rheumatic diseases (IRDs) that perform self-monitoring in daily clinical practice is still quite low.[11] In this article, we share our experiences with how we educated and motivated our patients with IRDs to participate in a self-monitoring program.

TOOL REUMANET

To stimulate patients in their self-management behavior, a digital tool can be helpful in which the patient can monitor and manage his or her disease outcomes. For this purpose, we developed at the department of Rheumatology of Bernhoven, a teaching hospital in Uden, The Netherlands, Reumanet Bernhoven. This is an online 2-factor authentication protected-personal health environment with several functions to support patients with IRD in their self-management behavior. This online personal health environment is available for the patient and the rheumatologist, but also the nurse, general practitioners, and/or physiotherapist can have access (with permission of the patient). The online personal health environment includes all patient characteristics, questionnaires, graphical overviews, lifestyle advices, and feedback opportunities, which include e-health modules and other relevant information adjusted for the individual patient with an IRD. This information is summarized in the dashboard (**Fig. 1**).

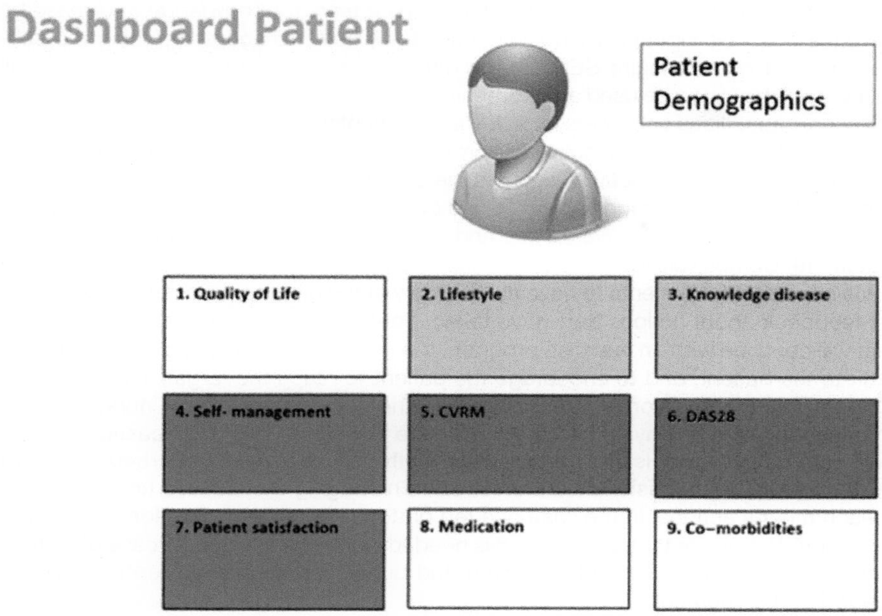

Fig. 1. Example of a personalized dashboard for patients in Reumanet. Green button: under control, no action needed. Red button: not under control, further action is needed. CVRM, cardio vascular risk management.

In more detail, first, patients can find an overview of their current and past medicines and blood values. Second, a monitoring function is available to track patients' disease activity. Patients can complete PROMs in this online system as preparation for the consultation with the rheumatologist and these scores are displayed in a graph. The patients can choose from scores such as the Rheumatoid Arthritis Disease Activity Index (RADAI) and the Rheumatoid Arthritis Impact Disease activity (RAID). These PROMs have shown to correlate well with objectively assessed measures and have good psychometric properties. In case the disease activity according to these PROMs and together with the patient set, exceeds a predetermined threshold, an alert appears in the online system. This enables identification of patients whose disease activity is not in line with the target and who might need further medical attention. Third, patients can self-add measurements of body weight or blood pressure and the results are also visible in a graph. Fourth, a chat function is available to send messages to health professionals. Last, patients can make use of the educational part of the program, called the library, which contains several leaflets and videos with information about various topics including information about their disease, medication use, fatigue, or working with RA.

PERSONALIZED DASHBOARD

For the different health professionals involved in the management of IRD, it is mandatory to have an overview of the status of the different domains of disease management (see **Fig. 1**). For example, the personalized dashboard contains the following domains: (1) *Quality of life*, in which different questionnaires will be filled in by patients about their current quality of life. (2) *Lifestyle factors*, such as physical activity behavior, smoking status, and diet of the patient will be followed over time. (3) *Knowledge of disease* by the patient will be inquired by questionnaires. (4) *Self-management*, using the self-management questionnaire SEMAS, the different domains of self-management will be measured that can be used as a screening instrument for nurses to assess patients' individual capabilities or barriers for self-management. (5) *Cardiovascular risk management (CVRM)*, the cardiovascular risk profile of the patient will be checked at least once a year. (6) *Disease activity*, such as the DAS28 in patients with RA, will be monitored. (7) *Patient satisfaction* and perceived quality of rheumatology care will be asked by questionnaires. (8) *Medication use* and adverse events will be documented in the system. (9) *Comorbidities*.

It is important for patients to have an overview of the disease process as well and to get feedback about actions they have taken. For instance, to make sure that the patient will continue with an exercise program, it is important to set a target, to give feedback to the patient, and to encourage the patient to reach the target. Therefore, it is important that in addition to the patient and the rheumatologist, the nurse, general practitioners, and/or physiotherapist also have access to this Web-based program (only with patient permission). In this way, both the patient and the rheumatologist and other health professionals are involved in managing the disease and are aware of each other's actions. In the case of a red button, the health professional or the patient should be aware that some action is needed in that domain. In the case of a green button, that domain is recently checked and under control and no further action is needed at this moment.

EDUCATION

To increase the number of patients participating in the self-management program, education of both the patients and the health professionals is important. Next to leaflets in the waiting room and general educational meetings, instruction classes have been organized to give patients a general instruction on how to use Reumanet. Patients can call or e-mail the help desk in case of any additional inquires. The staff at the outpatient clinic is also available to assist the patients in case they are needed before or after their visit to the rheumatologist.

CHANGING ROLE OF HEALTH CARE PROFESSIONALS

The introduction of a self-management outpatient clinic has, in addition to patients, also had consequences for the health care professionals. It requires a different approach, instead of the usual, old-fashioned paternalistic relationship, the role of the health care professional has changed to one in which the patient is coached to manage his or her disease. Different skills are required for this role, for instance motivational interviewing to help stimulate the patients to take their disease management role. For this purpose, a training program has been developed in which patients, health care professionals, and students learn together by exchanging experiences, knowledge, and skills.[12]

SELF-MANAGEMENT OUTPATIENT CLINIC

The traditional approach to monitoring IRD patients 2 to 4 times a year to assess disease activity is no longer necessary or appropriate but should be tailormade. As long as remission is not reached, frequent assessments need to be done to adapt the medication according to the Treat to Target guidelines. When the disease is under control, these measurements can be done less frequently and even remote self-monitoring would be feasible. Remote control by self-monitoring might also give important information about the disease course between outpatient clinic visits, as it has been shown that this information might have an important impact on the outcome of the disease. Therefore, self-monitoring in IRDs as a first step toward personalized health care enables patients as well as health care providers to get insights into the disease activity course over time.

In November 2017 we started with a "self-management outpatient clinic" to find if the monitoring frequency of patients can be decreased to 1 visit a year. Patients with IRDs are included if they fulfill the following inclusion criteria: (1) the patient is in remission or has low disease activity, (2) is motivated to take part in the self-management program, and (3) is able to use Reumanet. After consent, the patient receives information about (1) the aim of the self-management program and how to use Reumanet, (2) what the patient can expect from the health professionals, and (3) how to contact the outpatient clinic in case of questions. At the start, the self-management screening questionnaire is filled out by the patients to get to know if the patient encounters barriers in self-management behavior.[13] If appropriate, these barriers are solved before the start of the program or, in case this is impossible, the patients will not be included.

The patients can choose to track their disease activity by filling in the RAID or RADAI questionnaire. Patients can decide by themselves the frequency to fill in the RAID, for example, every week or every month. The results of the questionnaires are shown in a graph together with the DAS28 values performed by the health professional at the outpatient clinic visits (**Fig. 2**). To manage their disease, it is essential for them to perform self-management behavior: they need to remind themselves to fill in the questionnaire multiple times and based on the insight they gain in the graph and the preset target, they need to decide when to make an in-between appointment for a visit to the outpatient clinic. After 1 year, the rheumatologist and patient will evaluate the participation with a questionnaire to assess the patient's satisfaction.

FIRST RESULTS

By November 2017, 1125 patients with an IRD were already active in Reumanet Bernhoven. The degree to which patients make use of Reumanet Bernhoven differed

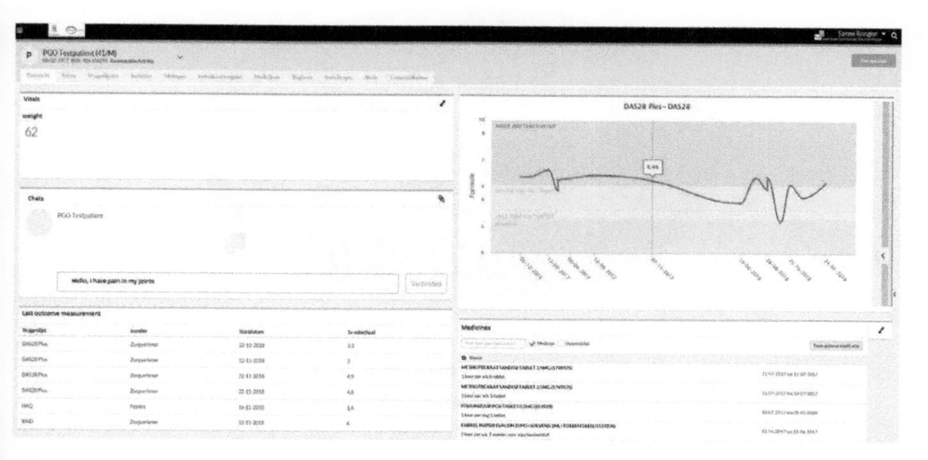

Fig. 2. Current Dashboard.

widely, and depended on patient needs, abilities, and skills. The results of Reumanet Bernhoven showed that 70% (n = 790) of the patients used it at least once a year, but only 13% (n = 100) of the patients used the self-monitoring tool. The remaining patients (n = 335) were questioned for not using Reumanet at home. The most common reason for not using Reumanet was not having a computer or e-mail address or the patient did not want to use a digital environment at home (**Fig. 3**). To increase the chance that patients are using the self-monitoring tool, it is important that they find useful information in this digital environment and therefore it is important to involve patients in the development of such a tool. It is also important to teach patients how to use it; to enhance continuous usage, patients need to receive feedback about it from their health care professionals at the outpatient clinic visits. Therefore, to increase the usage of Reumanet, the program will be continuously optimized and extended in accordance with patients' support needs and preferences. Earlier research shows that the patients' input is essential in the development of online tools[14,15] and that patients have various educational support needs.[16–18] To assess patients' support needs and preferences regarding the educational part of the online tool in our patient population, patients filled out a questionnaire with questions about their usage and their opinion about optimizing the content of the program. For instance, patients were asked what kind of functions should be added to Reumanet (eg, a newsletter, informational texts, or instructional videos). Also, patients were asked about which topics should be dealt with in the program (eg, new treatment options, the influence of nutrition on IRD, or medication usage).

Reasons Given by Patients for Not Using Reumanet

The first results (n = 35) showed that patients have several informational needs regarding physical impairments (pain, fatigue, and stiffness), and their treatment (how to prepare a visit to the outpatient clinic, improve their communication with health professional, usage of medicines, and being up to date on the newest treatment options). Informational texts, more graphical overviews, newsletters, instructional videos, and exercises should be added as functions to support patients in their

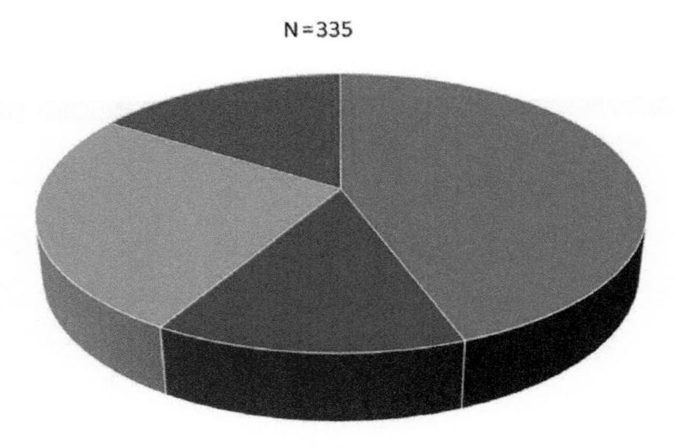

Fig. 3. Reasons Given by Patients for Not Using Reumanet. PHE, personal health environment.

informational needs. In addition to the questionnaire, we will conduct qualitative interviews to explore what patients exactly want; for instance, what kind graphical overviews they may want and which topics should be discussed in newsletters. Based on the results of the questionnaire and qualitative interviews, program material will be developed and added to the program to provide patients support in their self-management.

EXPERIENCES OF PATIENTS

The following quotes are from one of the patients who participated in the self-management program from the beginning of the program:

> *After the diagnosis of rheumatoid arthritis (RA) was made, my biggest fear for the rest of my life was to be dependent on others, but nothing is less true. I am using Reumanet, on which I regularly fill out questionnaires. I do that at home at a time that suits me. I determine the frequency myself, the moment and the time, no pressure from outside or a planned "quarter of an hour" in the hospital where it has to be done. I have direct insight into my medication, laboratory results, a library full of useful information, and there is room to add personal matters. Data from completed questionnaires are immediately processed and displayed in graphs that are readable and clear to me. The diagrams show progressive information in which I can set the period for which I want to look back.*

> *All of this really gives me the feeling of being in control of my own life and I don't feel myself a patient anymore but a human being. Meanwhile, I take the initiative to adjust the medication myself, of course under supervision and with the permission of my rheumatologist. If the disease activity values remain below the predefined target level, I don't plan a visit to the outpatient clinic. Because I only use a consultation with the rheumatologist when it is necessary, I can reduce the visits to the hospital to the minimum.*
> *Since last year, I go to the hospital much more often than before I had RA, but not as a patient but to help others how to deal with it. With this I have given it a place, accepted and enjoy the nice things in life despite my chronic disease.*

EXPERIENCES OF HEALTH CARE PROFESSIONALS

For the health care professional, the self-management program has changed the character of the outpatient visits significantly. Sometimes patients will start the consultation with a proposal to change their treatments based on their outcomes. The health care professional will discuss the pros and cons of the proposal with the patient and a truly shared decision will finally be made. Of course, there is a wide range in the degree of self-management between the different patients, similar to a visual analogue scale it can vary from a situation in which the health care provider decides alone, to a situation in which the patients tells the health care professional what he or she decided. It is a continuous learning process for both the patients and health care professionals, and because of this, the discussions during the outpatient clinic become more and more well matched.

SUMMARY

Currently in the management of patients with chronic diseases, more attention is being given to the patients' ability to adapt and self-manage their disease. The consequence of this is a change in the relationship between health care professional and patient: from a paternalistic to a shared decision approach. Currently the percentage of patients with chronic disease who practice self-management is still quite low. The rising health care costs and the decreasing number of available health care professionals in the near future compels us to find solutions in the short term. It would be very helpful if we are able to increase the percentage of patients who can manage and monitor themselves. In this respect, the following aspects are important takeaways:

- An easy to understand electronic health record with a well-organized dashboard informing both the patient as well as the health care professional about the status of the different health domains
- Attention should be paid to educate patients as well as health care professionals
- Use one electronic system for both the patient and health care professional
- The health care professional should discuss with the patient the results of the self-management and self-monitoring process.

REFERENCES

1. Tountas Y. The historical origins of the basic concepts of health promotion and education: the role of ancient Greek philosophy and medicine. Health Promot Int 2009;24(2):185–92.
2. Huber M, Knottnerus JA, Green L, et al. How should we define health? Br Med J 2011;343.
3. Silman AJ, Newman J, MacGregor AJ. Cigarette smoking increases the risk of rheumatoid arthritis. Results from a nationwide study of disease-discordant twins. Arthritis Rheum 1996;39(5):732–5.
4. Saevarsdottir S, Wedren S, Seddighzadeh M, et al. Patients with early rheumatoid arthritis who smoke are less likely to respond to treatment with methotrexate and tumor necrosis factor inhibitors: observations from the Epidemiological Investigation of Rheumatoid Arthritis and the Swedish Rheumatology Register cohorts. Arthritis Rheum 2011;63(1):26–36.
5. Saag KG, Cerhan JR, Kolluri S, et al. Cigarette smoking and rheumatoid arthritis severity. Ann Rheum Dis 1997;56(8):463–9.
6. Ajeganova S, Andersson ML, Hafstrom I, et al. Association of obesity with worse disease severity in rheumatoid arthritis as well as with comorbidities: a long-term followup from disease onset. Arthritis Care Res (Hoboken) 2013; 65(1):78–87.
7. Metsios GS, Stavropoulos-Kalinoglou A, Treharne GJ, et al. Disease activity and low physical activity associate with number of hospital admissions and length of hospitalisation in patients with rheumatoid arthritis. Arthritis Res Ther 2011;13(3): R108.
8. van Riel P, Alten R, Combe B, et al. Improving inflammatory arthritis management through tighter monitoring of patients and the use of innovative electronic tools. RMD Open 2016;2(2):e000302.
9. Hendrikx J, Fransen J, van Riel PL. Monitoring rheumatoid arthritis using an algorithm based on patient-reported outcome measures: a first step towards personalised healthcare. RMD Open 2015;1(1):e000114.
10. Stevenson FA, Cox K, Britten N, et al. A systematic review of the research on communication between patients and health care professionals about medicines: the consequences for concordance. Health Expect 2004;7(3):235–45.
11. Volpp K, Seth Motha N. Patient engagement survey: improved engagement leads to better outcomes, but better tools are needed. NEJM Catal 2016.

12. Vijn TW, Wollersheim H, Faber MJ, et al. Building a patient-centered and interprofessional training program with patients, students and care professionals: study protocol of a participatory design and evaluation study. BMC Health Serv Res 2018;18(1):387.
13. Eikelenboom N, Smeele I, Faber M, et al. Validation of Self-Management Screening (SeMaS), a tool to facilitate personalised counselling and support of patients with chronic diseases. BMC Fam Pract 2015;16:165.
14. Swift JK, Callahan JL. The impact of client treatment preferences on outcome: a meta-analysis. J Clin Psychol 2009;65(4):368–81.
15. Menon D, Stafinski T. Role of patient and public participation in health technology assessment and coverage decisions. Expert Rev Pharmacoecon Outcomes Res 2011;11(1):75–89.
16. Zuidema R, van Gaal B, Repping-Wuts H, et al. What is known about rheumatoid arthritis patients' support needs for self-management? A scoping review. Ann Rheum Dis 2014;73:1194.
17. John H, Hale ED, Treharne GJ, et al. 'Extra information a bit further down the line': rheumatoid arthritis patients' perceptions of developing educational material about the cardiovascular disease risk. Musculoskeletal Care 2009;7(4):272–87.
18. Radford S, Carr M, Hehir M, et al. 'It's quite hard to grasp the enormity of it': perceived needs of people upon diagnosis of rheumatoid arthritis. Musculoskeletal Care 2008;6(3):155–67.

Mobile Apps for Rheumatoid Arthritis

Opportunities and Challenges

Elizabeth Mollard, PhD[a], Kaleb Michaud, PhD[b,c,*]

KEYWORDS

- Mobile applications • Rheumatoid arthritis • Self-management • Mhealth
- Smartphone

KEY POINTS

- Mobile apps allow patients with rheumatoid arthritis (RA) to monitor, manage, and share information about their disease with their rheumatologist on a regular basis.
- Although health-related apps for other chronic conditions are an established market with growing use, RA-related apps are still in their early stages of development and adoption.
- Barriers to the growth of mobile apps for RA include a limited evidence base, technology infrastructure, and patient hand disability among others.

INTRODUCTION

Mobile device applications have great potential to improve health outcomes in individuals with rheumatoid arthritis (RA). RA and other rheumatic and musculoskeletal diseases (RMDs) affect patients in a myriad of ways throughout their daily lives, most commonly through pain and decreased physical function. Health-related quality of life dimensions have been measured by patient-reported outcomes (PROs) and accelerometers in research and by patients for many years; however, now these data can be collected easily by a mobile device. In general, mobile-collected data are stored in a mobile application (app), which is either kept on the device itself or shared to a cloud-based portal where patients and clinicians can review the information.

There are a variety of health-related applications that can aide in self-monitoring, motivational support, behavioral feedback, health information education, and even

---

Disclosure Statement: Dr K. Michaud receives grant funding from the Rheumatology Research Foundation.

[a] College of Nursing, University of Nebraska Medical Center, 550 North 19th Street #357, Lincoln, NE 68588, USA; [b] Division of Rheumatology and Immunology, University of Nebraska Medical Center, 986270 Nebraska Medical Center, Omaha, NE 68198-6270, USA; [c] FORWARD, The National Databank for Rheumatic Diseases, Wichita, KS, USA

* Corresponding author. 986270 Nebraska Medical Center, Omaha, NE 68198-6270.

E-mail address: kmichaud@unmc.edu

Rheum Dis Clin N Am 45 (2019) 197–209
https://doi.org/10.1016/j.rdc.2019.01.011 rheumatic.theclinics.com
0889-857X/19/

care delivery. Engaging with a health-related app has been proposed to change an individual's health beliefs and behaviors,[1] build knowledge and skills in self-management of health,[2] enhance self-efficacy to manage symptoms,[3] decrease health risk behaviors,[4] and lead to improved clinical outcomes.[5,6] In addition to the benefits of engaging with apps, current mobile devices incorporate several powerful tools with the potential to measure and track objective health information with minimal effort from the patient.[7] These features include GPS, accelerometers, gyroscope, and magnetometer, which can track human movement, activity, and sleep on mobile apps.

The existing shortage of rheumatologists is predicted to worsen over the next decade, while simultaneously the demand for rheumatology care is expected to increase.[8] Empowering patients to be active participants in their RA disease management through mobile applications has the potential to improve medication adherence and symptom management, reduce disease activity, and increase the number of necessary in-person visits. Because RA is an individualized disease with distinct personal triggers for symptoms, mobile apps offer the benefit of being accessible at any time and in any location where a patient can access their device. Carrying a mobile device at all times and using it in public places is now an accepted cultural norm, with 9 out of 10 individuals reporting almost never being without their device.[9] Therefore, there are seemingly few reasons a patient could not actively or passively collect data about their RA symptoms and management strategies throughout their day using these same devices. Collecting RA-related information can help the patient learn more about their disease and its management, and this information can be shared with their rheumatologist to optimize decision-making at in-person clinical visits.

Nearly 325,000 health-related apps are available, with 78,000 added between 2016 and 2017.[10] Yet, the market for RA health-related apps is still in its infancy.[11] The purpose of this article is to discuss opportunities and challenges associated with RA-related mobile apps along with some of the authors' experiences using them for research, clinical practice, and personal health improvement. Researchers interested in both RA and non-RA RMDs should find value from these experiences.

TYPES OF MOBILE APPLICATIONS FOR RHEUMATOID ARTHRITIS

Mobile health-related apps have many different purposes. The number of apps specifically for RA is limited but growing. Here, several different categories of apps that can be used for RA are outlined (**Table 1**).

Patient Education

RA patient education apps may include general information about RA, medications, disease management, and important health care resources available to patients with RA. Fifty-eight percent of smartphone users have downloaded a health-related app, often for the sole purpose of gathering health information.[12] Luo and colleagues[11] (2018) found that 25% of the apps available for RA were exclusively patient education. The benefits to educational apps are that they provide essential information available to the patient at any time. Educational apps may be especially important for patients who are newly diagnosed with RA or who are currently having a flare of RA and desire immediate answers. The downside of this type of application is that education alone has been shown to do very little to improve health outcomes in chronic illness.[13] In addition, after initial use of the app, there is unlikely to be continual engagement because once information is obtained there is little motivation to return to the app on a regular basis. Finally, an education-only app offers little more than a consolidated

Table 1
Types of apps for patients with rheumatoid arthritis and their limitations

Mobile Application Type	Description	Limitations	Examples Available in 2019
Patient education	Provide information on rheumatoid arthritis and disease management	• Limited use • Education alone unlikely to improve patient outcomes	• ArthritisID (Arthritis Consumer Experts) • Rheumatoid Arthritis Treatment (Creative Live Apps)
Clinician tool	Clinical measurements, such as DAS, HAQ, Clinical Reference	• Unlikely to improve patient outcomes	• RheumaHelper (Modra Jagoda) • DAS Calculator (Greg Fiumara) • RAVE (DKBmed LLC)
Self-management	Measure variables, such as pain, medication use, sleep, mood, stiffness, diet, etc.	• Requires technology proficiency • Requires ongoing engagement with the app • Reporting fatigue	• Arthritis Power (Jeffrey Curtis), • LiveWithArthritis (eTreatMD), • TRACK and REACT (Arthritis Foundation)
Passive monitoring	Monitoring of behaviors through mobile device use, GPS, accelerometer, weather, etc.	• Newest technology with limited apps available • Limited variables that can be measured • May require additional wearables	• No RA or RMD related found Other examples • RADAR Passive RMT (The Hyve) • Ginger.io (company no longer using passive sensing)
Apps with gamification	Either add-on element or stand-alone app with gameplay element (rules of play, points, competition, etc) to improve RA	• No rheumatology apps in this space according to authors' knowledge • Research gap in negative elements of gamification	• No RA or RMD related found Other examples • Charity Miles • Pokémon Go (Niantic, Inc.)
Telemedicine	Rheumatologists meet with the patient over HIPAA-compliant app platform to deliver care	• Changes patient/ physician rapport • No physical touch • Cannot collect clinician joint count or tender points	• No RA or RMD related found Other examples • Doctor on Demand • Teladoc • MDLive

version of a web-based search result, which a patient is also able to perform on a mobile device if they have a wireless connection.

Educational apps highlight a common issue with mobiles apps in general—apps should be viewed primarily as a tool. With the view of apps as a tool, it can be seen that if patients will not or do not use it or even have access to it, it cannot help them. Translating a Website or a book to an app moves it into a different format in the hopes of it becoming more accessible. If the content was not valuable before it was placed in an app, it will not become more useful just because it is presented in app format. On the other hand, apps offer the opportunity to optimize educational experiences with hands-on videos, animations, and other media that may be best used in this format along with possibly a more customized-to-the-user experience.

Clinician Tool Apps

Eighty-seven percent of physicians own a smartphone or tablet, and it is assumed that these statistics are similar for rheumatologists.[14] Most of the physicians use a medical related app. There are several rheumatology professional clinician tools available in the mobile app format, which include apps containing an individual tool or apps containing a "toolbox" of tools including disease activity scales and calculators, diagnostic criteria, and other rheumatic disease reference information. Clinician mobile apps offer a close-at-hand mobile tool for providers to use as needed throughout their clinical day. These apps enhance the experience of the rheumatologist by organizing information and tools and potentially improving the time spent on clinical visits (**Fig. 1**). Clinician-based apps are designed to improve clinical visits, and little research has been conducted as to how they may improve the outcomes of the individual with RA. Another consideration is that many clinicians use specific tools that are already incorporated into their electronic health record system. Therefore, the uses of clinician-based apps have the potential to duplicate the effort of the clinician or are simply redundant with tools already available within the electronic health record.

Self-management Apps

Self-management apps for RA can allow for a patient to collect individual data such as daily recording of pain, times of medication administration, food diaries, imaging of the hand,[3] and other features to allow a patient to monitor the state of their disease. A significant benefit to patients engaging in self-management is that they become active in their own care. Instead of using recall to report their symptoms and experience to their rheumatologist once every 3 to 6 months at their regular appointments, they come with detailed knowledge about their individualized disease and treatment experience

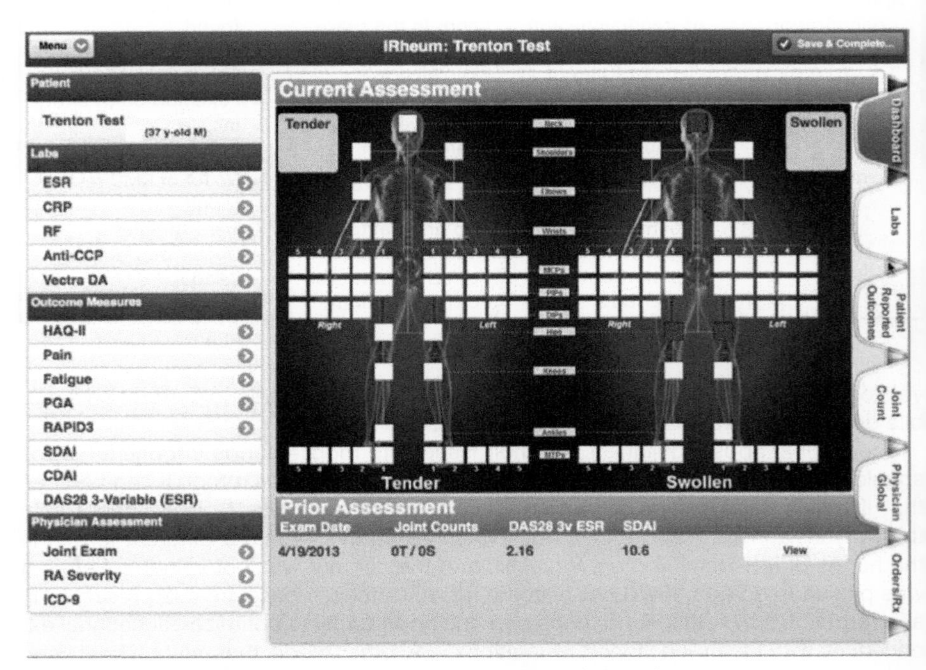

Fig. 1. iRheum tablet-based app to improve recording of clinical measures.

recorded regularly over time, improving the time spent with the rheumatologist for strategizing their care going forward. Clinicians can view these self-obtained records to gather information on treatment compliance and point out patterns that may be related to increased disease activity. There are limitations to using self-management apps, such as challenges in getting enthusiastic patients to regularly engage with the app or that patients become tired of regularly recording their information day in and day out.

In a research, the authors studied a self-management app with novel optical imaging technology.[3] Patients (n = 34) photographed their hand once per month that was analyzed to note changes in the anatomy of the hand. Patients also entered daily information about their RA experience such as pain levels, diet, and treatments (**Fig. 2**). Common to mobile app use in general, there was a significant dropout rate of 38% (13 of the 34) over 6 months.[15] The authors were able to interview all but one participant who dropped out of the intervention group to learn more about what

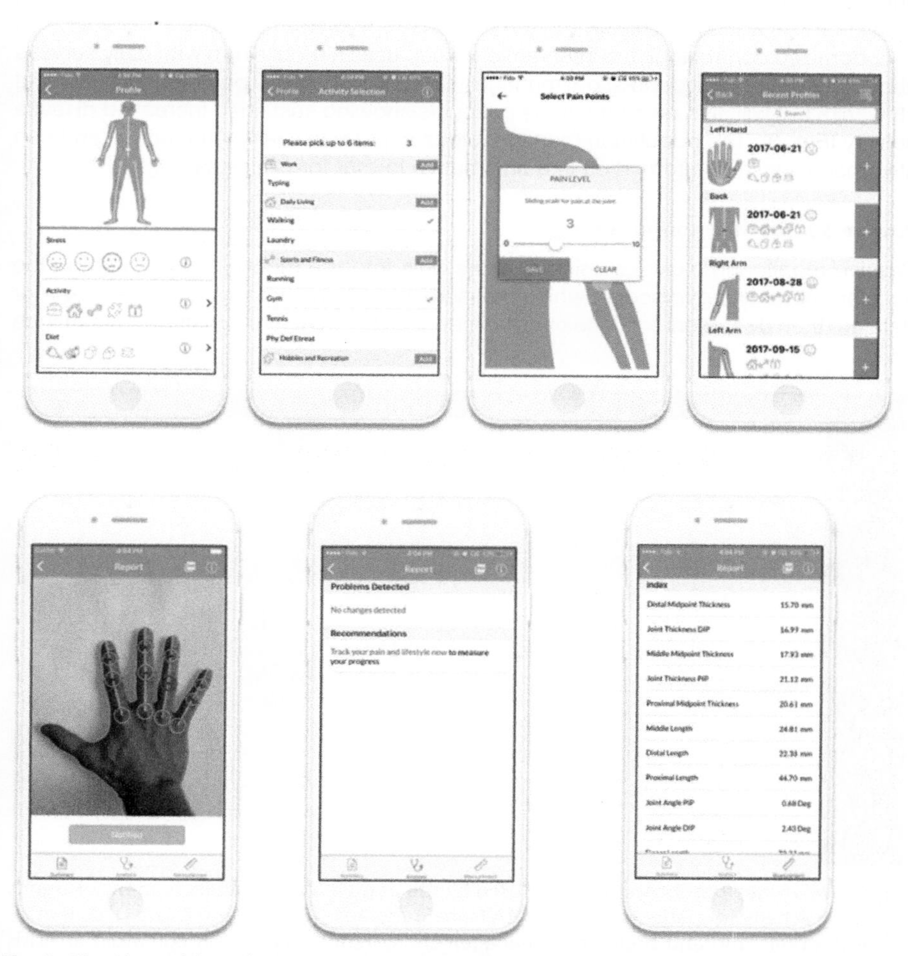

Fig. 2. The Live With Arthritis app allows patients to track information about their RA and changes to their hand using a novel optical imaging feature.

barriers existed that prevented them from using the app more regularly. The common themes were frustration with technology, that RA hand disability made the app difficult to use and that some participants preferred their current self-management system. Although the authors like the idea of a unique app with optical imaging, if a pen and paper tool is going to help a patient better self-manage their disease, then that may be the system that will work for that patient. The benefit for those participants who finished the study was an increase in self-efficacy in managing symptoms as measured by the Patient-Reported Outcomes Measurement Information System Self-Efficacy Managing Symptoms questionnaire (Intervention 2.80 vs Control −1.66, $P = .04$) and trends toward improved clinical outcomes. The challenges of app use reminded us that sometimes an app is just the tool a patient needs to take charge of their RA. For researchers and clinicians, the authors wonder how they can design and encourage them to use the tool and benefit from it.

Although many apps offer the option to share data with the patient's rheumatologist, the amount and usefulness of data could make sorting through this information onerous for the clinician. One way this has been remedied is represented in an ongoing study that has added a clinically trained person to serve as a population manager.[16] In a randomized control trial, the intervention group uses a mobile app with daily surveys about their RA. The population manager checks in with all participants at 6 and 18 weeks but will also reach out if the patient is showing sustained increased disease activity (**Fig. 3**). The population manager aides in potential early intervention and can also make sense of information in a summative format for clinicians.

Passive Sensor Monitoring Apps

Passive monitoring includes using sensors built into the mobile device such as the accelerometer and gyroscope, which measure movement, activity, and sleep. Sensor data are then documented alone or combined with the patient's subjective experience

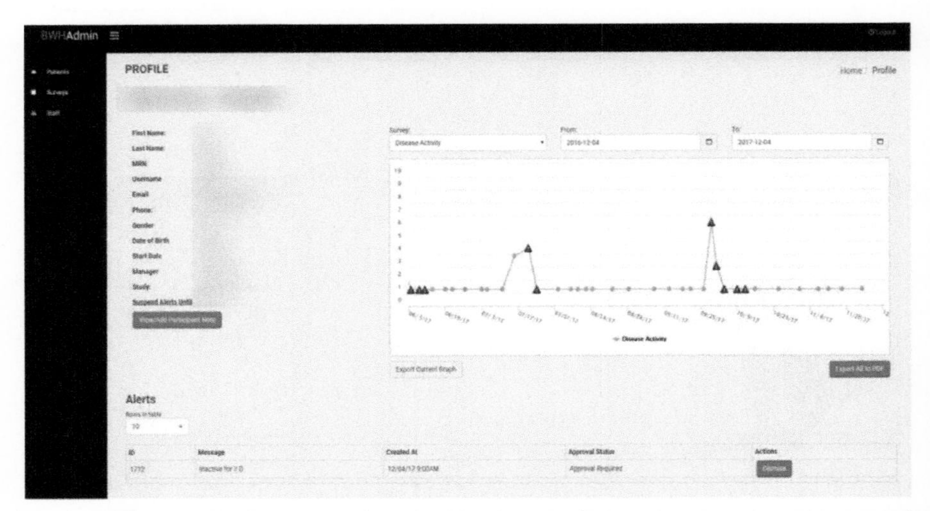

Fig. 3. Web-based dashboard interface used by the population managers to monitor trends in disease activity for patients using the RA Flare Study App. (*From* Wang P, Luo D, Lu F, et al. A novel mobile app and population management system to manage rheumatoid arthritis flares: protocol for a randomized controlled trial. MIR Res Protoc 2018;7(4):e84. Available at: https://www.researchprotocols.org/2018/4/e84/.)

to gain more insight into disease activity. The GPS function, which measures the patient's location, can be synced to information such as the weather, humidity, pollen counts, or smog in the same GPS location to identify potential flare triggers. Some apps come with or require adding a wearable such as a smartwatch, temperature sensor, or electrocardiogram band to gather data. The major benefit to passive measurement is that the patient does not grow fatigued of gathering data and is not burdened by the process.

In other chronic disease studies, passive measurements have shown that sedentary behavior, how little the patient moves the phone, and more minutes using the screen on functions of the mobile device may be associated with greater symptom severity.[17] The limitations include the accuracy and usefulness of the data collected for persons with RA. Although passive monitoring may have the potential to highlight bad days with severe symptoms using activity-based data, the RA-specific measures such as stiffness and pain generally must include a subjective experience that may not be feasible with current passive sensor technology.

In a study to determine if passively collected digital measures could predict PRO measures in patients with rheumatic diseases, the authors found that moving averages of text length was associated with pain and moving averages of mobility were associated with patient global, HAQ-II and PAS-II.[18] RA flares were also associated with moving averages of mobility radius. This study showed that there was good adherence to recording daily/weekly symptoms and disease activity that coordinated with passive measures, opening up opportunities for further, larger studies.[19]

Apps with Gamification

Gamification is using a game or competitive element to motivate patients to use the features of an app. For example, an app focused on medication adherence may give a reward for each medication that is taken on time as prescribed; this may be a simple scoring mechanism such as earning a virtual badge or could include apps that promote earning real-life monetary benefit. Charity Miles is an app that allows the user to earn money for their favorite charity by being physically active. Gamification is primarily a motivator for behavior change, although a gaming app targeted at patients with RA but unrelated to collecting disease information is potentially feasible.

One gamification feature called augmented reality shows promise for health-related applications. Augmented reality is an interactive experience where actual real-life experiences are augmented by an electronic device to add an augmented component that is not real to life. An example would be the game Pokémon Go that involves movement unrelated to the goal of fitness. Participants aim to collect augmented reality characters (Pokémon) either at specific locations determined by geolocation or by hatching them by traveling 2 to 10 km and by doing so engage in physical activity and gameplay. Pokémon Go gameplay (which one of the authors uses regularly) has been shown to be associated with increased physical activity and improved daily function and psychosocial wellbeing.[20–22] Gamification with augmented reality is an example of using a gaming app that could improve health without directly focusing on a health problem or goal—the most popular games in this area require physical activity and often reward either steps/running or hand motions. There are few chronic illness health-related apps in existence that have a gamification element, and this space seems to be wide open for rheumatology.

Telemedicine Apps

Telemedicine allows for the delivery of rheumatology care via video chat for live clinical sessions using the camera on the mobile device or an asynchronous store and forward system such as what is used for radiographic interpretation. Benefits include improved access to care for individuals in rural and remote locations and those with limited transportation. Limitations of an app focused on rheumatology telemedicine include the absence of physical touch, which creates difficulty in a hands-on specialty where joint count and tender points are critical. In addition, patients with RA are often in significant pain much of their time and appreciate the human touch of an experienced rheumatologist. Rheumatologists and patients alike appreciate the rapport of in-person visits. At the time of publication, there was no rheumatology-specific telemedicine application in the Apple or Google app store, although there are general telemedicine apps and web-based services that a rheumatologist could choose to use. Rheumatology services in the telemedicine space have primarily been used to communicate with the patient and work with a health professional with the patient to act as a proxy for the in-person rheumatologist. Much of this is limited by technology and the ability to be reimbursed for the visit consultation. Telemedicine for rheumatology in both the app format and otherwise is discussed by E. Michael Lewiecki and Rachelle Rochelle's article, "Project ECHO: Telehealth to Expand Capacity to Deliver Best Practice Medical Care," in this issue and elsewhere.[23]

CHALLENGES TO USING MOBILE APPS FOR RHEUMATOID ARTHRITIS

Technology Barriers

The use of a mobile health app for RA requires a consistent and reliable individual mobile device, in addition to a functioning network infrastructure presenting multiple layers of potential technical barriers to deliver the preferred app experience. Although access to smartphone and tablet technology is more common than ever, infrastructure to support consistent mobile technology use is still relatively limited in rural areas.[24,25] Rural patients with RA are one of the populations with the greatest need for further health services due to their distance from qualified rheumatologists and may be additionally limited by factors such as internet connection or 3G/4G cellular network service. Although it seems like a problem that should be easily remedied, the costs associated with placing this infrastructure to distant and remote places is high, and few stakeholders are advocating for these changes compared with urban areas. These factors have made the technical barriers of mobile apps the most significant in areas that may benefit from them the most.

In addition to infrastructure, a large technology barrier is the hardware or actual physical devices for app use. There are a seemingly endless number of devices on the market. In 2015, there were more than 25,000 different types of Android devices alone.[26] The variation in individual device hardware and operating system (eg, Android, iOS) makes it difficult to ensure universal app functionality. Whenever the app needs an update, which is frequently because of updates to operating systems, developers must retest and validate the app, and once approved, there are almost certainly additional unexpected issues that require additional updates. Screen size, graphics capacity, and sensor and hardware capabilities (eg, accelerometer, gyroscope) vary for each device, making it difficult to find one app that will provide the same experience after factoring in all these variables.[27] Although it has been shown that allowing patients to use their own device may increase engagement with apps[28] use in both research and clinical settings, relying on individual mobile device presents inconsistency due to variance in data plans, Wi-Fi services or mobile provider coverage areas, screen size, operating system (eg, Android vs iOS) and condition of the mobile device.

Evidence Base of Mobile Apps for Rheumatoid Arthritis

Despite the large number of health-related apps available, the Food and Drug Administration reviews only about 20 per year.[29] The use of specific mobile applications has a limited evidence base due to the fast-moving pace of technology and the slow pace of research funding and further delays in publishing results in peer reviewed scientific journals. Although research can highlight whether the use of any mobile health application improves outcomes, the evidence base for a specific app is difficult to determine. When beginning a study using mobile apps, researchers must determine whether they want to test a preexisting application or develop an application from scratch, which adds significant costs and time to the research. Although software development tools exist, such as iOS ResearchKit, you are limited to only using Apple or you will have to find an equivalent system in Android, meaning you will find difficulty in creating a uniform app with the same functionality. Once the app of study has been determined, changes that occur due to ongoing required updates to the hardware and software affect the intervention treatment fidelity.

Another research consideration is the device itself. Researchers can provide a smartphone to participants to increase the uniformity of the experience of each participant. However, it is not guaranteed that participants will use the provided device as their primary smartphone or tablet, if at all. Providing a physical device adds significant costs to the research budget, and use of the patient's own device may increase engagement and use of the app because the individual is likely already comfortable using the device. Another potential option is for researchers who provide devices to take the extra step of moving contacts and the participants' SIM card to ensure the research device becomes the primary device, although most smartphone users have preferences on which device they would like to use (eg, Android vs iOS). Beyond the costs of providing a device, once a smartphone device is provided there are other considerations that can become potential problems, such as the amount of time a participant is provided the device, how to handle the need for an upgraded device, what service/data plan is provided, and problems with broken devices.[30]

By the time a study is published on a mobile application for RA, it is unknown whether the evidence will apply to the current version of the app and if it will be universal to all smartphone device users outside of a research setting. The lack of consistent evidence base creates a barrier for clinicians to use or recommend an app to patients with RA.

For example, in 2004, a study was conducted using Palm Personal Digital Assistants (PDAs) where patients were asked to track pain and function 3 times per day. At the time this was revolutionary technology and patients were motivated to use it. In a follow-up study with no tech observations, nearly all benefits of the PDA intervention disappeared, resulting in a publication on the Hawthorne effect.[31] The Hawthorne effect is a behavioral change that is observed in study participants that may modify their behavior based on the perception of being observed. This study was a good example of challenges in keeping up with ever-changing technology, because PDAs were completely out of use at the date of that publication, as well as some of the potential limitations of mobile app-based research where participants may believe they are being observed and therefore behave differently than they would if they were choosing to use an app or technology on their own.

Patient Barriers

Patients with RA are a unique population to mobile health technology because they are more likely to have pain and disability in their hands compared with other chronic illness–affected populations. Hand pain and disability present limitations for the actual operation of mobile devices. One potential way to still gain benefit from an app includes offering mobile apps that include passive measurements of health where the participant may only need to place the device in their pocket. In addition, apps designed for RA should include voice-enabled technology where symptoms such as pain score or stiffness can be recorded based on the patient speaking in the values. In a study using an optical imaging technology for hand monitoring on a self-management app, the authors found that participants with more severe RA of the hand had difficulty using the camera without recruiting help.[3] Although this was a barrier in this study, even camera functions could be voice enabled in future app versions.

Another challenge can be the technical ability of the patient. Mobile apps are more widely adopted in the general adult population than by older adults, and the challenges with mobile app adoption and continued use tend to increase with age.[32] One factor related to age and app adoption is how much the individual desires to integrate technology into their daily life. RA diagnosis increases with age and most patients in the United States with RA are older than 65 years.[33] Many older adults are interested in using mobile apps, but studies have shown that older adults prefer only to use technology when they can quickly see the benefits of using the app with ease and shortly after initial use.[34] If benefits are not obvious and frustration is felt with initial use, older adults tend to cease using the app altogether.[35]

Another major concern for patients is the privacy and security of their health information. Although companies have created safeguards to protect the privacy and security of patient health data, the possibility of health data being breached from a mobile app is possible.[36] Many mobile apps operate as a personal app and not a HIPAA-compliant protected space for health information. Patients may not know the difference, and clinicians may not know the differences when recommending a specific app. In addition, individuals who keep other private information such as bank records on their computer or mobile device may be concerned that downloading a new app for health may breach other information that is already on the mobile device. Many individuals who feel hesitant about the safety and security of their information will choose to opt out of mobile app technology for managing their health.[37]

Patients who currently have a self-management system that is working for them, such as the use of pen and paper logs, or who have low disease activity may be uninterested in a mobile app for their RA.[3] Although mobile app technology presents great opportunities for patients, not all patients will feel that the technology is useful for them. In addition, most patients with RMDs have additional important health conditions that would not likely be captured in an RMD-specific app.

SUMMARY

Mobile devices and apps have created much excitement in both the tech and health care industry. Although there is a growing market for mobile apps related to chronic disease management and care, the development and use of RA-related apps is still in its early stages of growth.

There are a variety of types of apps that can be used for RA, including those for patient education, clinician tools, self-monitoring, passive monitoring, apps with gamification, and telemedicine apps. An important note to keep in mind about all of the app possibilities is that mobile apps are tools. In order to work to make meaningful change for the individual with RA, the app must deliver something useful to the patient, whereas simply putting something in app format is unlikely to make a tool useful. With that caveat, providing a tool at the fingertips of patients that works and may improve their health or wellbeing has the potential to be life-changing. It is important to find what tools and approaches deliver value for patients with RA first and foremost and then strategize ways to bring those tools to patients in app format.

An important limitation of all mobile apps is that technology is constantly changing. Currently, mobile apps are in a stage of rapid growth and development. In recent history, there was excitement about PDAs. Although it already seems that mobile apps are longer lived than PDAs, it is important to remember that mobile apps are not necessarily a permanent fixture. Again, app creation must be focused on delivering helpful tools designed with functional features, many of which would be useful even without mobile technology.

Self-management seems to us to be one of the most valuable uses of mobile app technology. With the technology in the hands of patients, they can record daily symptoms and treatment information that can easily be organized, graphed, and shared with clinicians. Although patients can do the same system with pen and paper, it does seem that mobile apps have the potential to optimize this experience. When combining self-management with a population manager as in Wang and colleagues,[16] clinical time spent with rheumatologists can be maximized and patients may have decreased disease activity and improved outcomes. Adding passive measures and gamification may further improve the self-management experience and usefulness of collected data.

In summary, mobile apps create a great opportunity to improve care and disease management for patients with RA. There is a limited evidence base as to what mobile apps work and why they work along with challenges in guaranteeing intervention fidelity when studies are conducted. Despite this it seems mobile apps are an important fixture for both patients and clinicians dealing with RA. It is an exciting time for the development and use of mobile apps and the forward-moving use of technology for RA management and care.

REFERENCES

1. Zhao J, Freeman B, Li M. Can mobile phone apps influence people's health behavior change? an evidence review. J Med Internet Res 2016;18(11):e287.
2. Bashi N, Fatehi F, Fallah M, et al. Self-management education through mhealth: review of strategies and structures. JMIR Mhealth Uhealth 2018;6(10):e10771.
3. Mollard E, Michaud K. A mobile app with optical imaging for the self-management of hand rheumatoid arthritis: pilot study. JMIR Mhealth Uhealth 2018;6(10):e12221.
4. Iacoviello BM, Steinerman JR, Klein DB, et al. Clickotine, a personalized smartphone app for smoking cessation: initial evaluation. JMIR Mhealth Uhealth 2017;5(4):e56.
5. Hui CY, Walton R, McKinstry B, et al. The use of mobile applications to support self-management for people with asthma: a systematic review of controlled studies to identify features associated with clinical effectiveness and adherence. J Am Med Inform Assoc 2017;24(3):619–32.
6. Chow CK, Redfern J, Hillis GS, et al. Effect of lifestyle-focused text messaging on risk factor modification in patients with coronary heart disease: a randomized clinical trial. JAMA 2015;314(12):1255–63.
7. Lowe SA, Ólaighin G. Monitoring human health behaviour in one's living environment: a technological review. Med Eng Phys 2014;36(2):147–68.

8. Battafarano DF, Ditmyer M, Bolster MB, et al. 2015 American College of Rheumatology workforce study: supply and demand projections of adult rheumatology workforce, 2015-2030. Arthritis Care Res (Hoboken) 2018;70(4):617–26.
9. Rainie L, Zickuhr K. Chapter 1: always on connectivity. Pew Research Center Report; 2015.
10. Research2guidance .mHealth Economics 2017 – current status and future trends in mobile health. Available at: https://research2guidance.com/wpcontent/uploads/2017/11/R2G-mHealth-Developer-Economics-2017-Status-And-Trends.pdf. Accessed November 3, 2018
11. Luo D, Wang P, Lu F, et al. Mobile apps for individuals with rheumatoid arthritis: a systematic review. J Clin Rheumatol 2018. https://doi.org/10.1097/RHU.0000000000000800.
12. Krebs P, Duncan DT. Health app use among US mobile phone owners: a national survey. JMIR Mhealth Uhealth 2015;3(4):e101.
13. Bodenheimer T, Lorig K, Holman H, et al. Patient self-management of chronic disease in primary care. JAMA 2002;288(19):2469–75.
14. Ventola CL. Mobile devices and apps for health care professionals: uses and benefits. P T 2014;39(5):356–64.
15. Localytics. Mobile apps: whats a good retention rate?. 2018. Available at: http://info.localytics.com/blog/mobile-apps-whats-a-good-retention-rate. Accessed November 3, 2018.
16. Wang P, Luo D, Lu F, et al. A novel mobile app and population management system to manage rheumatoid arthritis flares: protocol for a randomized controlled trial. JMIR Res Protoc 2018;7(4):e84.
17. Low CA, Dey AK, Ferreira D, et al. Estimation of symptom severity during chemotherapy from passively sensed data: exploratory study. J Med Internet Res 2017; 19(12):e420.
18. Michaud K, Pedro S, Schumacher R. Can passively-collected phone behavior determine rheumatic disease activity? [abstract]. Arthritis Rheumatol 2018; 70(suppl 10). Available at: https://acrabstracts.org/abstract/can-passively-collected-phone-behavior-determine-rheumatic-disease-activity/. Accessed November 3, 2018.
19. Rainie L, Zickuhr K. Americans' Views on Mobile Etiquette. Washington, DC: Pew Research Center; 2015. Available at: http://www.pewinternet.org/2015/08/26/americans-views-on-mobile-etiquette/.
20. Howe KB, Suharlim C, Ueda P, et al. Gotta catch'em all! Pokémon GO and physical activity among young adults: difference in differences study. BMJ 2016;355: i6270.
21. Tateno M, Skokauskas N, Kato TA, et al. New game software (Pokémon Go) may help youth with severe social withdrawal, hikikomori. Psychiatry Res 2016;246: 848–9.
22. LeBlanc AG, Chaput JP. Pokémon go: a game changer for the physical inactivity crisis? Prev Med 2017;101:235–7.
23. E. Michael Lewiecki and R Rochelle. Project ECHO: telehealth to expand capacity to deliver best practice medical care. [Epub ahead of print].
24. Duncombe R. Mobile phones for agricultural and rural development: a literature review and suggestions for future research. Eur J Dev Res 2016;28(2): 213–35.
25. Nandi S, Thota S, Nag A, et al. Computing for rural empowerment: enabled by last-mile telecommunications. IEEE Commun Mag 2016;54(6):102–9.

26. Open signal. Android fragmentation. Available at: https://opensignal.com/reports/2015/08/android-fragmentation/. Accessed November 3, 2018.
27. Hurt CP, Lein DH Jr, Smith CR, et al. Assessing a novel way to measure step count while walking using a custom mobile phone application. PLoS One 2018; 13(11):e0206828.
28. Ben-Zeev D, Schueller SM, Begale M, et al. Strategies for mHealth research: lessons from 3 mobile intervention studies. Adm Policy Ment Health 2015;42(2): 157–67.
29. US Department of Health and Human Services, Food and Drug Administration. Mobile Medical Applications: Guidance for Industry and Food and Drug Administration Staff. Available at: http://www.fda.gov/downloads/MedicalDevices/DeviceRegulationandGuidance/GuidanceDocuments/UCM263366.pdf. Accessed February 9, 2015.
30. Jacobson J, Lin CZ, McEwen R. Aging with technology: seniors and mobile connections. Can J Comm 2017;42(2):331–57.
31. Wolfe F, Michaud K. The Hawthorne effect, sponsored trials, and the overestimation of treatment effectiveness. J Rheumatol 2010;37(11):2216–20.
32. Kruse CS, Mileski M, Moreno J. Mobile health solutions for the aging population: a systematic narrative analysis. J Telemed Telecare 2017;23(4):439–51.
33. Hunter TM, Boytsov NN, Zhang X, et al. Prevalence of rheumatoid arthritis in the United States adult population in healthcare claims databases, 2004-2014. Rheumatol Int 2017;37(9):1551–7.
34. Matthew-Maich N, Harris L, Ploeg J, et al. Designing, implementing, and evaluating mobile health technologies for managing chronic conditions in older adults: a scoping review. JMIR Mhealth Uhealth 2016;4(2):e29.
35. Wildenbos GA, Peute L, Jaspers M. Aging barriers influencing mobile health usability for older adults: a literature based framework (MOLD-US). Int J Med Inform 2018;114:66–75.
36. Martínez-Pérez B, de la Torre-Díez I, López-Coronado M. Privacy and security in mobile health apps: a review and recommendations. J Med Syst 2015;39(1):181.
37. Navarro-Millan I, Zinski A, Shurbaji S, et al. Perspectives of rheumatoid arthritis patients on electronic communication and patient-reported outcome data collection: a qualitative study. Arthritis Care Res (Hoboken) 2019;71(1):80–7.

Patient-Reported Outcomes Measurement Information System Versus Legacy Instruments

Are They Ready for Prime Time?

Vivian P. Bykerk, MD

KEYWORDS

- PROMIS • Patient-reported outcome measurement information system
- Legacy patient-reported outcome measurements
- Patient-reported outcome measures • Rheumatic diseases • Item response theory

KEY POINTS

- The National Institutes of Health–funded Patient-Reported Outcomes Measurement Information System (PROMIS) uses self-reports to evaluate and monitor physical, mental, and social well-being.
- Unlike Legacy PROs, PROMIS measures can be implemented across diseases, and use a common T-score metric-based scoring system derived using item response theory.
- PROMIS has been validated in 3 rheumatic diseases, for use in research and practice.
- PROMIS measure scores can predict scores of Legacy PROs (called cross-walking) and can be the only set of measures needed to assess PROs.

INTRODUCTION

Measurement of patient-reported health status is a critical element in assessing a patient's well-being. Self-reports inform the diagnostic process, medical decision making, and monitoring of clinical status, treatment effects, and response. The use of validated patient-reported outcome measures (PROs) are relatively new to the study and practice of rheumatology, with most having been developed over the past 2 decades. In research settings, PROs are intended to capture health domains that cannot be easily measured through clinical observation, or laboratory or imaging tests. Only patients can report on their subjective experience of symptoms and functional issues, medication effects, and how these affect their lives. Although the integration of PROs into clinical research is now standard practice, the use of PROs in settings of care is still in flux, with ongoing debate as to what measures or instruments to use and in an

Disclosures: Consultant for Amgen, Pfizer, Sanofi/Genzyme, Scipher, UCB.
The Hospital for Special Surgery, Inflammatory Arthritis Center, Weill Cornell Medical College, 535 East 70th Street, New York, NY 10022, USA
E-mail address: bykerkv@hss.edu

Rheum Dis Clin N Am 45 (2019) 211–229
https://doi.org/10.1016/j.rdc.2019.01.006
rheumatic.theclinics.com
0889-857X/19/

era of electronic health records (EHRs), how this can be best accomplished in terms of feasibility, utility, and interpretation.

LEGACY PATIENT-REPORTED OUTCOMES

Legacy PROs have strengths and limitations (**Box 1**). Most were developed for specific health conditions, using classic test theory (CTT) for scoring algorithms. Validation or field testing was limited to restricted populations. Legacy PROs assessing the same health domains use varying items, variable structure of questions, with different anchors and scoring ranges. Lack of standardization of scores among instruments measuring the same construct across studies in the same disease limits the ability to perform meta-analyses of data from studies.[1]

Legacy PROs have mostly been completed on paper forms, stored in paper charts. When needing to assess multiple domains, several Legacy PROs were often required to assess all domains of interest. However, many include similar items phrased in different ways, which would frustrate, confuse, or burden patients. To date, few Legacy PROs have been incorporated into EHR systems with concomitant paper

Box 1
Benefit and limitations of Legacy patient-reported outcomes (PROs)

Rationale for Continued Use of Legacy PROs

Familiar; scores have meaning to clinicians and patients

Disease specific, or common to diseases within specialty area

Some are easy to administer when responses are paper recorded

Some widely adopted/entrenched in clinical practice (ie, Routine Assessment of Patient Index Data 3 [RAPID III])

Many have items with good content validity; were used to develop PRO Measurement Information System (PROMIS) item banks

Some are generic to multiple diseases/rheumatic diseases (eg, Short Form 36 [SF36])

Limitations of Legacy PROs:

Limited generalizability: many specific for 1 domain in 1 disease

More than 1 Legacy PRO to measure the same domain or health construct: variable outcome measures among studies

When combining Legacy PROs, similar items can be confusing and impact responses (eg, time frame: today vs past week vs past 6 months)

Leads to high questionnaire burden if using multiple Legacy PROs at once

Missing data may invalidate the PRO

Items/Questions can be ambiguous, irrelevant, or meaningless (eg, taking a tub bath is irrelevant to many)

Floor and ceiling effects evolved as patient characteristics changed from original derivation of the Legacy PRO

Few generic Legacy PROs can be used across diseases, most have user fees

Inconsistent presentation of items can reduce reliability (ie, item anchors switch within same tool)

Unnecessary number of items inefficient (eg, if patient can walk 2–3 miles and get out of car or train, no need to ask if they can get out of a chair)

administration creating documentation challenges. Evolution of disease characteristics and more effective interventions have resulted in new floor or ceiling effects for some Legacy PROs previously validated in populations with different characteristics. Until this past decade, frequently used nonspecific Legacy PROs to assess health-related quality of life (HRQoL), such as the Short Form 36 (SF36), Health Utilities Index 3 (HUI-3), and the EuroQol 5D (EQ5D), have been used in rheumatology, but their implementation has been limited by low reliability and licensing costs.[2] These generic measures are difficult to score and do not measure all domains in a way that is relevant or always comprehensible for patients. However, large datasets of Legacy PROs used over decades are available for validation of new PROs in development.[3] Currently only Legacy PROs are accepted to measure a patient's perspective in clinical trials. Some, such as the Routine Assessment of Patient Index Data 3 (RAPID III)[4] are widely integrated into practice settings, have high relevance and meaning to providers, are familiar to patients, and are viewed by many as being the "gold standard" for PRO measures. Thus, transitioning away from using specific Legacy PROs will require a shift in mindset, research methods with convincing evidence to do so.

There is a need for a system of self-assessment in which health domains and constructs can be similarly assessed using items and short forms tested using psychometric methods to assess domains common to multiple conditions. Improvements in efficiency (fewer items to complete), flexibility (use of interchangeable items), and precision (providing estimates with low measurement error) of revised items would lower the burden for patients providing self-assessments in research or practice. Using instruments that cover core domains important to patients and that inform health status is key to expanding the use of PROs in research and practice, and to improve patient-centered care.

WHAT IS PATIENT-REPORTED OUTCOMES MEASUREMENT INFORMATION SYSTEM?

The PRO Measurement Information System (PROMIS) comprises a set of person-centered health measures compiled using state-of-the-art psychometric methods based on item response theory (IRT).[5] PROMIS facilitates self-assessment of the 3 World Health Organization–defined core pillars of health (physical, mental, and social well-being). PROMIS was developed as part of the National Institutes of Health Roadmap to develop a means to assess PROs using metrics that could be applied across conditions and disease states, irrespective of the diversity of individuals being assessed in a precise, reliable, and efficient fashion.

The PROMIS system consists of item banks of questions, many adapted from Legacy PROs, to assess symptoms and perceptions about performance for 7 profile domains of health most relevant to people living with chronic health conditions or illness. These include physical function, pain interference and impact, fatigue, sleep disturbance; emotional health, including depression, anxiety, and the ability to participate in social roles (**Fig. 1**).[6] Item banks assessing additional PROMIS domains have been added over the past 10 years (see **Fig. 1**). Each item bank can assess multiple facets of a health domain associated with 1 of the 3 pillars of health and well-being.

THE HISTORY AND DEVELOPMENT OF PATIENT-REPORTED OUTCOMES MEASUREMENT INFORMATION SYSTEM

Work to conceptualize PROMIS, construct item banks, and develop a computer adaptive testing system (CATs) intended to efficiently assess domains using a minimum number of relevant, patient-endorsed items by taking advantage of IRT occurred between 2004 and 2014. By taking advantage of psychometric methods and

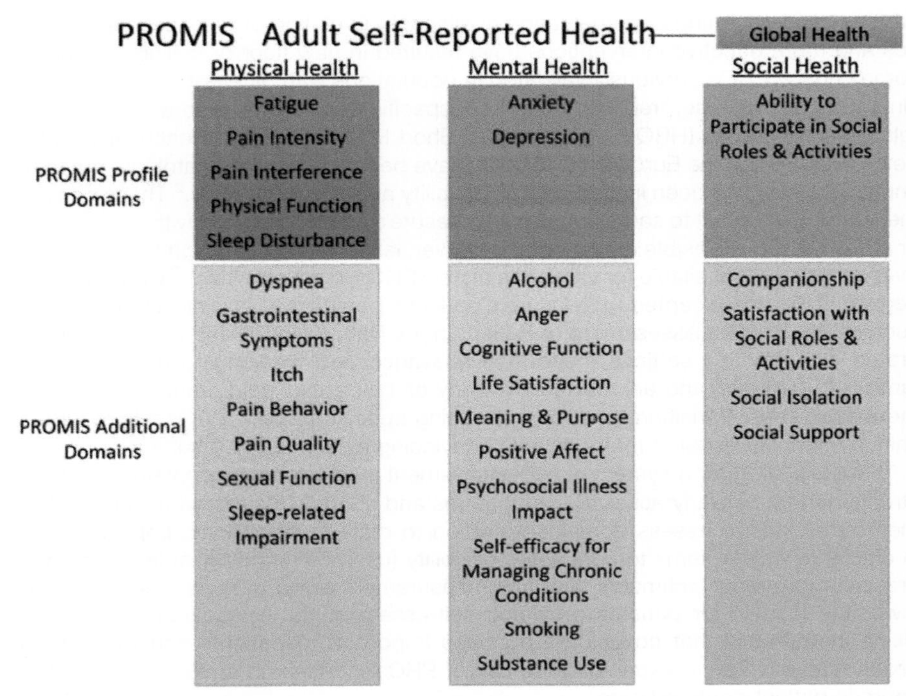

Fig. 1. Seven core item banks that assess PROs are included as PROMIS profile. Item banks assessing additional health domains linked to 1 of 3 core pillars of health. (*Courtesy of* PROMIS Health Organization, Evanston, IL. PROMIS is a registered trademark of the Department of Health and Human Services. © 2008–2018; with permission.)

advances in measurement science, the PROMIS development team used a structured and orderly process to develop each item bank that would assess a core health domain (**Fig. 2**). The series of steps started with defining each health construct and domain, identifying items, and constructing item banks informed by qualitative and mixed method studies (**Table 1**)[7](REF change Terwee Text). IRT was used to compile related items that could be calibrated to a T-score metric that could predict a score for each trait of interest.[8]

Initially, 14 item pools were identified and tested in both the US general population and clinical groups, using an online panel and clinic recruitment. A scale-setting subsample was created reflecting demographics proportional to the 2000 US census.[9]

Eleven item banks and a 10-item Global Health Scale were then calibrated based on responses from a normative sample of 21,133. Short forms for each bank were developed. Construct validation included comparison of each short form with the overall bank, and with other well-validated and widely accepted ("Legacy PRO") measures. Short forms were intended for use in situations when all available items assessing a health domain cannot be administered using a CATs. Item banks were released when following initial validation including demonstration of good reliability across most of the score distributions in people with varying health conditions and illnesses.

Overall, 45,000 people contributed data to the PROMIS system; 1500 contributed to qualitative research and 35,000 to quantitative research (including 25,000 adults and 10,000 children) providing data to calibrate measures and develop reference norms. Spanish PROMIS items were validated by 4000 Spanish-speaking participants.[9]

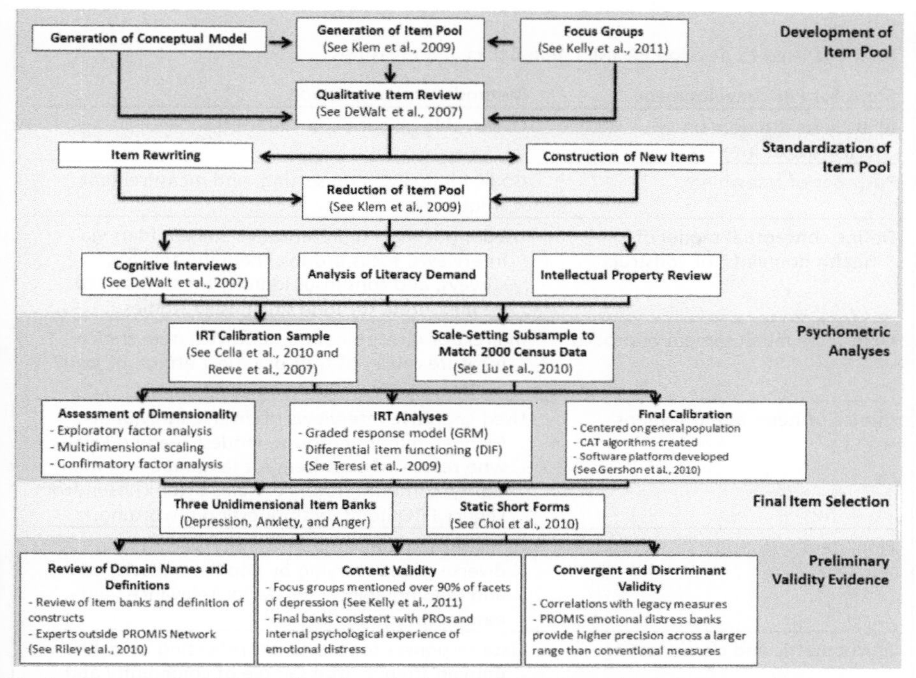

Fig. 2. An example of the order of methods used by PROMIS developers to derive a psychometrically sound and valid item bank to assess a health domain. (*From* Choi SW, Schalet B, Cook KF, et al. Establishing a common metric for depressive symptoms: linking the BDI-II, CES-D, and PHQ-9 to PROMIS Depression. Psychological Assessment 2014;26(2):513–27.)

Additional validation has continued over the past 5 years across different conditions and diseases to demonstrate generic applicability of the new item banks.

ADMINISTERING PATIENT-REPORTED OUTCOMES MEASUREMENT INFORMATION SYSTEM ITEM BANKS

Item banks were constructed for flexible use. Each comprises 4 to 10 items. If implemented using the CATs, domain scores are calculated immediately and efficiently predict scores according to a T-score metric. CATs algorithms present a minimal number of items without compromising reliability or precision; however, each person may not respond to the same items depending on their health status for that domain. Health outcomes can be assessed using validated short forms chosen from domain-specific item banks, CATs, or as multidomain profiles of measures (**Fig. 3**). PROMIS measures are validated to include a fixed set of 4, 6, or 8 items grouped to assess the 7 core health domains (eg, PROMIS 29) (**Table 2**). Additional short forms (4–12 items) can assess additional domains.

PROMIS generic health measures were developed and validated to inform HRQoL for use in clinical research. These are available in multiple languages and validated for many diseases.[10] A shorter 10-item Global Health Scale (PROMIS-10) was developed for use as a health utility measure for economic studies. This enables self-report of overall health and physical well-being, and queries 5 domains (pain severity, social well-being, physical function, fatigue, and emotional health) using 1 to 2 general questions for each (**Table 3**).[11] Seven PROMIS Domains were used to develop a preference

Table 1
Methods used to develop PROMIS item banks and measures

Steps for PRO Development	Methods/Implementation
Identify health domain or construct of interest	Observable or not (ie, a "latent trait").
Purposes of assessment	Goals for assessment, setting, and measurement frequency.
Define conceptual model of health domain(s) or construct	Used input from representative stakeholders via interviews, focus groups, thematic analysis, surveys, and consensus identifying all facets to be measured, through qualitative studies.
Determine measurement approach	Indirect or direct measurement. Will item choice measure causes of trait or reflect effects of trait? Generate pool of potential items.
Choice of items and questions	Used cognitive interviews of diverse individuals (gender, minority groups, modest reading levels) who reviewed each item for language and item clarity, content relevance. Items often chosen from Legacy PRO items, with question rewording.
Final item selection	Items chosen met content validity; vetted by a diverse group (varying by gender, minority status, and reading ability) for clarity, relevance, and ease of interpretation.
Psychometric and classic testing	Data responses to item banks reflecting a health domain from a large sample of community and clinical participants were tested using CTT for factor structure. Full range of responses was used to calibrate and standardize a scoring system using IRT.
Assembly of item banks	Items reflecting domain of interest and full spectrum of functional or symptoms responses for a health domain were assembled into item banks.
Validation plan	Content validity (ie, face and construct validity, including correlation with Legacy PROs, and responsiveness to show meaningful change) and reliability planned and confirmed.
Expand item banks for use in multiple conditions	Test health domain in different diseases and multiple settings; reconfirm validity each time.
Calibrate items along a standardized metric	Items responses cover the full continuum of a standardized scale for measurement confirmed through iterative testing.

Abbreviations: CTT, classic test theory; IRT, item response theory; PRO, patient-reported outcome; PROMIS, PRO measurement information system.

Modified from Terwee CB, Crins MHP, Boers M, et al. Validation of two PROMIS item banks for measuring social participation in the Dutch general population. Qual life Res 2019;28(1):211–20; and *Data from* Cella D, Riley W, Stone A, et al. The patient-reported outcomes measurement information system (PROMIS) developed and tested its first wave of adult self-reported health outcome item banks: 2005-2008. J Clin Epidemiol 2010;61(11):1179–94; and HCW dV, CB T, LB M. Measurement in medicine: a practical guide (practical guides to biostatistics and epidemiology) 1st edition. 1st edition. Cambridge University Press; 2011.

scoring system (PROPr).[12,13] Summary scores were validated against generic based preference measures including the HUI and EQ5D.[14] The PROMIS-10, like the PROMIS 29, 43, and 54 profiles are freely available. Responses encompass those aspects of well-being valued by a person at a time in his or her life that is being influenced by a

Short Forms
• Subsets of item banks
• Focused on single domain
• Usually include 4–10 items
Computer Adaptive Tests
• Tailored electronic questionnaires
• Focuses on a single domain
• Items presented following initial item response aim to improve precision
• Usually 4–12 items
PROMIS Profiles or Measures
• Collection of short forms assess 7 core domains
• Profiles can have between 4–8 items for each domain

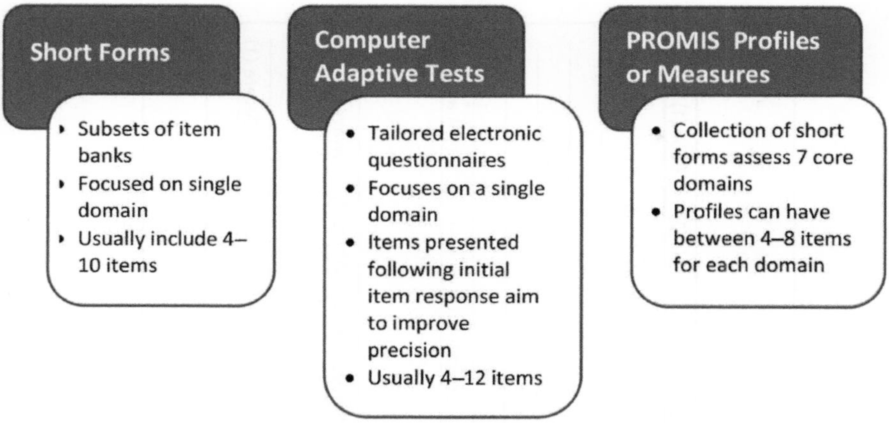

Fig. 3. PROMIS short forms, CATs, and profiles. Each health domain can be assessed using items from the item bank for that domain. Short forms may include all items or a subset for a domain. Use of the full set of items or a validated subset of items constitutes a PROMIS profile or measure. (*Courtesy of* PROMIS Health Organization, Evanston, IL. PROMIS is a registered trademark of HHS. © 2008-2018; with permission.)

health condition. A person's subjective state, values, social circumstances, age, and other factors will influence his or her perception, behaviors, and activities.

Until recently, HRQoL could be assessed only by using generic Legacy PROs, such as the SF36, SF12, HUI-3, and EQ5D. The PROMIS-10 and PROMIS 29 short forms can be used to assess value in health, usually measured using Legacy PROs without additional costs, and the PROMIS-10 can predict the EQ5D[11]. Work is ongoing to compare PROMIS Global Health Scores with Legacy generic measures currently regarded as standard in clinical trials.[14,15] Of note, items in the Global PROMIS-10 do not overlap with the PROMIS-29/43 or 57 profiles. Whether or not the Global-10 can be used interchangeably with these other PROMIS profiles requires further evaluation.

UNDERSTANDING PATIENT-REPORTED OUTCOMES MEASUREMENT INFORMATION SYSTEM SCORES

The PROMIS scoring system is grounded in IRT, which is used to calibrate raw scores from short forms to a corresponding location on a T-score metric (**Figs. 4** and **5**). The

Table 2
PROMIS profiles: PROMIS 29/43/57

		PROMIS Measures (Number of Items per Domain)		
	Health Domain	**PROMIS 29**	**PROMIS 43**	**PROMIS 57**
1	Anxiety	4a	+ 2a = 6a	+ 2a = 8a
2	Depression	4a	+ 2a = 6a	+ 2a = 8a
3	Fatigue	4a	+ 2a = 6a	+ 2a = 8a
4	Physical function	4a	+ 2a = 6a	+ 2a = 8a
5	Sleep disturbance	4a	+ 2a = 6a	+ 2a = 8a
6	Social roles and participation[a]	4a	+ 2a = 6a	+ 2a = 8a
7	Pain interference	0–10	0–10	0–10

[a] V 1.0 assesses satisfaction with social roles and participation; V 2.0 assesses ability to participate in these.

Table 3
PROMIS global 10

Global Items		Response Options				
Q 1–5, 9 Ask Patients to Rate Each Domain with Stem "In General"		Excellent (5)	Very Good (4)	Good (3)	Fair (2)	Poor (1)
Global01	… rate *your health*:	—	—	—	—	—
Global02	… rate *your quality of life*:	—	—	—	—	—
Global03	… rate *your physical health*:	—	—	—	—	—
Global04	… rate *your mental health*, mood, and your ability to think:	—	—	—	—	—
Global05	… rate your satisfaction with your social activities *and relationships:*	—	—	—	—	—
Global09	…rate how well you *carry out your usual social activities and roles.*	—	—	—	—	—
		Completely (5)	Mostly (4)	Moderately (3)	A little (2)	Not at all (1)
Global06	To what extent are you able to carry out your everyday *physical activities,* such as walking, climbing stairs, carrying groceries, or moving a chair?	—	—	—	—	—
		Never (5)	Rarely (4)	Sometimes (3)	Often (2)	Always (1)
Global10	How often have you been bothered by *emotional problems, such as feeling anxious, depressed, or irritable*?	—	—	—	—	—
		None (5)	Mild (4)	Moderate (3)	Severe (2)	Very Severe (1)
Global08	How would you rate your *fatigue* on average?	—	—	—	—	—
Global07	How would you rate your *pain* on average? (0 = no pain; 10 = worst pain imaginable)	0 1 2 3 4 5 6 7 8 9 10				

Items query general health (Q1, 2), mental health 2a (Q4, 10); physical health (Q3, 6), social health (Q5) and pain intensity (Q7).

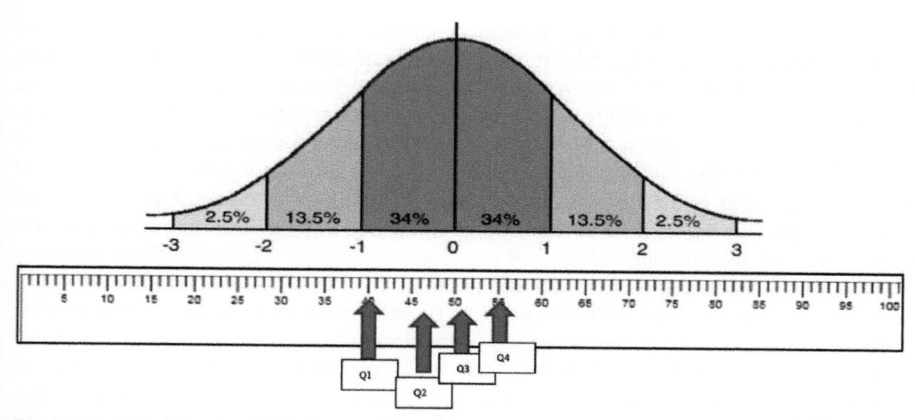

Fig. 4. Q1: Can lift groceries, if no difficulty. Q2: Walk for 15 min, if no difficulty. Q3: Do stairs at normal pace, if no difficulty. Q4: Can do 2 hours labor: no difficulty. Stop as of calibrated score will be 55.

range of scores reflects referent norms established using scores from a large normative data set and scores from people with chronic illnesses, and different contextual factors were used to established a comprehensive range of point estimates along this metric (range 0–100). As a result, PROMIS scores are standardized, interval level scales in which each 10-point deviation from the norm (midpoint of 50) represents 1 standard deviation (see **Fig. 4**). Ratings are devised so that higher scores mean more of that trait, whether desirable or not. Higher scores of symptom domains (eg, anxiety, depression, fatigue, pain interference, and sleep disturbance) indicate a score worse than the norm, whereas lower scores of a function or role (eg, physical function) indicate worse perceived ability.

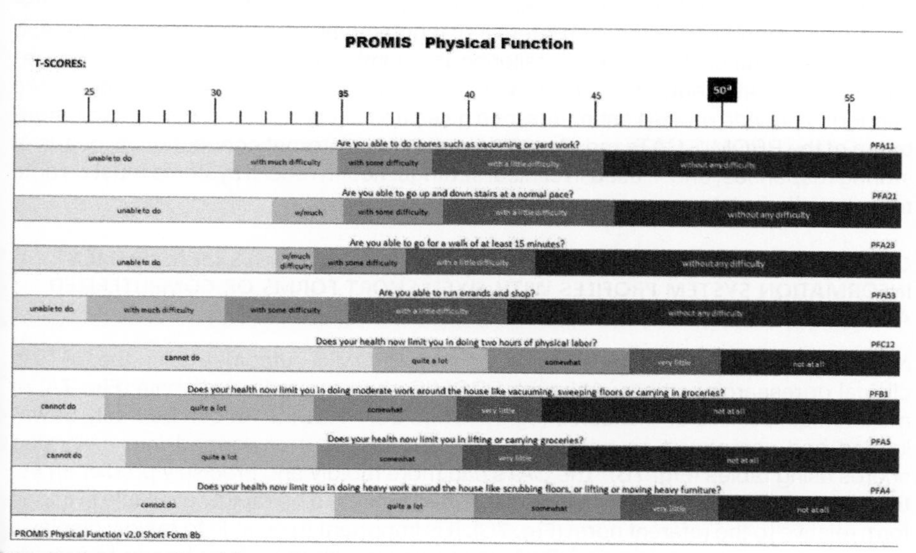

Fig. 5. An example of how items in the Physical Function Item Bank map to the PROMIS T-score metric. [a] A score of 50 = mean of general population reference sample. (*Courtesy of* PROMIS Health Organization, Evanston, IL. PROMIS is a registered trademark of HHS. © 2008-2018; with permission.)

By using IRT as an ordered response model, the mapping of response options from multiple items can ensure each item bank predicts all levels of a given trait or domain along the breadth of the T-score metric standardized scale. The CATs uses these IRT-based models to efficiently choose the fewest number of items (4–10) that most precisely predict an individual's score for a given trait. Thinking about physical function, if the answer to the first item about doing hard labor for 2 hours is yes, and the second response to doing chores is yes, then a few subsequent items will be chosen that map closely to this higher level of reported function (see **Fig. 4**). Scoring methods developed using IRT assume individuals will respond similarly for a given level symptom or ability for health domain, despite differences in health disparities or cultural beliefs.[16]

Thus, scores for a given domain reflect all possible responses to items sets for that domain, and a person's score reflects a prediction of that latent trait being assessed relative to the norm. PROMIS scores are really probabilities estimating a level of health status for that trait as it would map onto a precalibrated scale. In the example of the PROMIS Depression Short Form (**Fig. 6**), a PROMIS score of 60 would be equivalent to low moderate depression using older Legacy measures and a comparison between Legacy measures are possible.[17] In considering what a score of 60 means (ie, 2 standard deviations above the norm), **Fig. 6** demonstrates item responses that would correspond to this position along the T-score metric.

USING COMPUTERIZED ADAPTIVE TESTS TO COMPLETE ITEMS FOR HEALTH DOMAINS

IRT-calibrated item banks underlie the use of CATs algorithms. Item difficulty and responses can be thought of as being placed along a continuous ruler starting from least to highest. CATs will present the initial item to approximate an individual's approximate probable level of his or her latent trait. Depending on the first response, additional items help to determine a more precise level of the trait.[18] Although CATs may draw items from 1 or 2 item banks, the CATs requires fewer items to precisely estimate the probable level for each latent trait (unobservable health domain) of interest. As a system, the CATs is flexible, tailoring the number of required items to prior responses, and efficient, as only a few items from the larger item bank options are needed to provide precise estimates for a given trait of interest.[1] However, implementation of the PROMIS CATs mostly requires a reliable Internet connection, a means of storing responses, and, if used in clinical settings, health record systems must be able to include their data.

CONSIDERATIONS IN CHOOSING PATIENT-REPORTED OUTCOMES MEASUREMENT INFORMATION SYSTEM PROFILES WITH FIXED SHORT FORMS OR COMPUTERIZED ADAPTIVE TEST SYSTEMS

Not all have ready access to devices to capture PROMIS outcomes using the CATs in clinical or research settings. Although PROMIS short forms for 1 domain (**Fig. 7**A) or multidomain profiles or measures (eg, PROMIS 29, PROMIS 10) can be freely downloaded and completed on paper, raw scores must be transformed into calibrated scores using tables (**Fig. 7**B). The CATs can more rapidly and precisely predict an estimate for a trait, and software allows calibrated scores to be rapidly available in image form relative to the referent norm (**Fig. 7**C). It is important to be able to rapidly display a score as an image comparing an individual's score with the referent norm to provide the most accurate patient-level scores and changes for use in clinical care. The CATs are most suitable to foster rapid assessment of self-reported health that could result in more meaningful clinical encounters.[19]

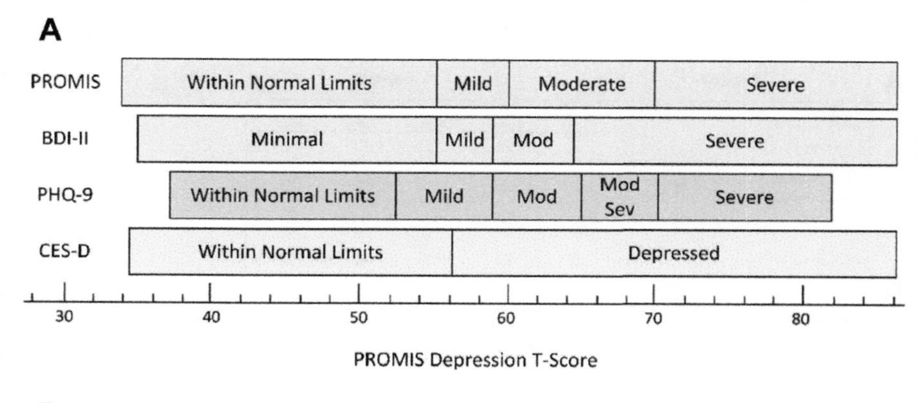

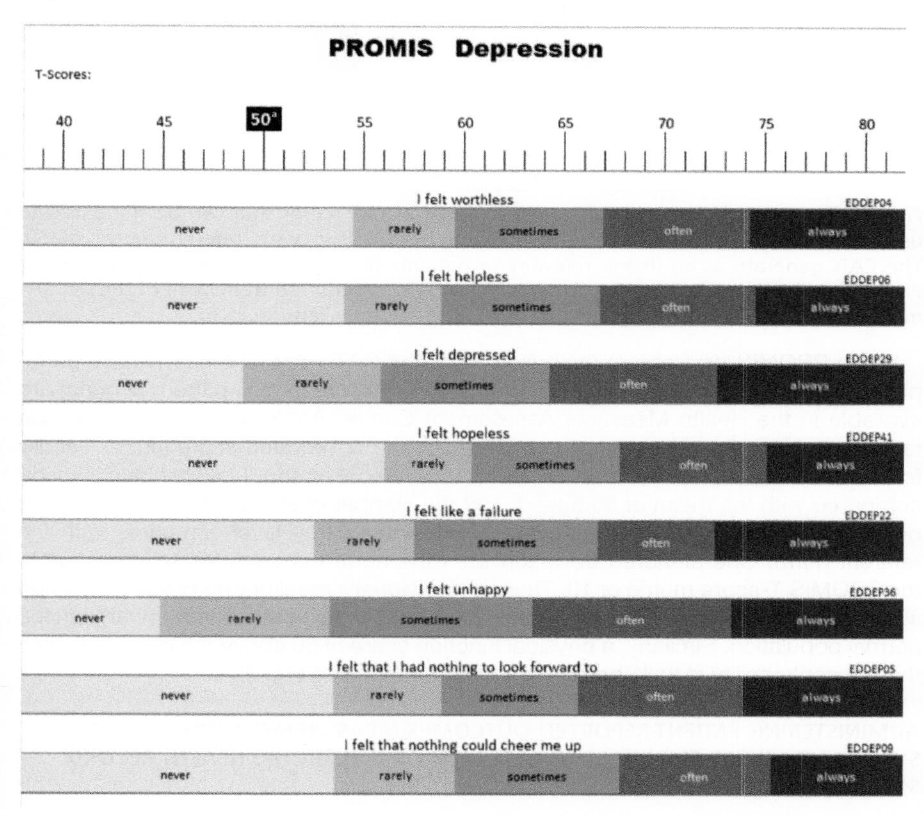

Fig. 6. (*A*) The relationship of Legacy PROs to PROMIS metrics using depression inventories as an example. (*B*) An example of PROMIS item responses and how they map onto the T-score metric. [a] A score of 50 = mean of general population reference sample. (*A*) and (*B*) provide an example of how Legacy PROs compare with PROMIS scores, suggesting how one Legacy score to predict other Legacy PRO scores within in the same health construct. BDI, Beck Depression Inventory; CES-D, Center for Epidemiologic Studies–Depression; PHQ-9, Patient Health Questionnaire 9. (*Data from* [*A*] Choi SW, Schalet B, Cook KF, et al. Establishing a common metric for depressive symptoms: linking the BDI-II, CES-D, and PHQ-9 to PROMIS Depression. Psychological Assessment 2014;26(2):513–27; and *Courtesy of* [*B*] PROMIS Health Organization, Evanston, IL. PROMIS is a registered trademark of HHS. © 2008-2018, with permission.)

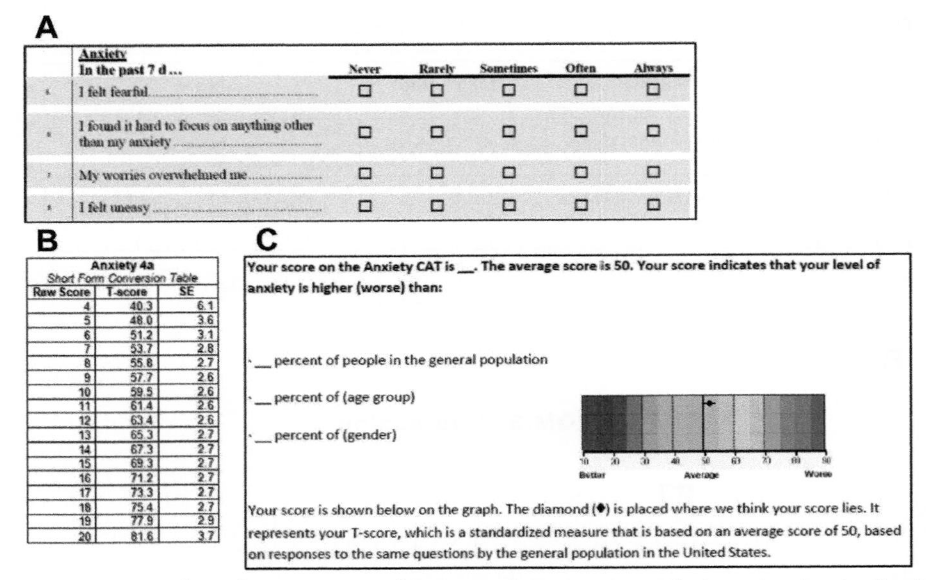

A

Anxiety In the past 7 d ...	Never	Rarely	Sometimes	Often	Always
I felt fearful	☐	☐	☐	☐	☐
I found it hard to focus on anything other than my anxiety	☐	☐	☐	☐	☐
My worries overwhelmed me	☐	☐	☐	☐	☐
I felt uneasy	☐	☐	☐	☐	☐

B

Anxiety 4a
Short Form Conversion Table

Raw Score	T-score	SE
4	40.3	6.1
5	48.0	3.6
6	51.2	3.1
7	53.7	2.8
8	55.8	2.7
9	57.7	2.6
10	59.5	2.6
11	61.4	2.6
12	63.4	2.6
13	65.3	2.7
14	67.3	2.7
15	69.3	2.7
16	71.2	2.7
17	73.3	2.7
18	75.4	2.7
19	77.9	2.9
20	81.6	3.7

C

Fig. 7. PROMIS short form responses (*A*) summed as raw scores that can be standardized using T-score metric from tables (*B*) allowing comparison with referent norm of 50. The CATs generate as an image relevant to patients (*C*). SE, standard error. (*Courtesy of* PROMIS Health Organization, Evanston, IL. PROMIS is a registered trademark of the Department of Health and Human Services. © 2008-2018; with permission.)

When PROMIS profiles are used instead of the CATs, raw scores must be transposed into a standardized score. Scoring tools (called response pattern scoring) are available in the Health Measures Assessment Center. Applicable score conversion tables can be used to translate the total raw score or prorated score into a T-score for each short form completed by individuals. Recalibrated T-scores and can be compared with the mean of 50 based, and the number of standard deviations that it deviates from the mean, informs how an individual's trait level compares with the referent norm. One standard deviation from the norm corresponds to a change in the PROMIS T-score metric of 10. Thus, an individual's recalibrated physical function score of 40 would be 2 one standard deviations below the norm or 34% lower than the normal population. Similarly, a physical function score of 60 above the norm indicates that person's ability is xx% better than most people (see **Fig. 4**).

ADMINISTERING PATIENT-REPORTED OUTCOMES MEASUREMENT INFORMATION SYSTEM MEASURES EMBEDDED IN RESEARCH OR ELECTRONIC HEALTH RECORD SOFTWARE

PROMIS measures can be administered electronically for specified health domains of interest using the PROMIS CATs via computer or tablet. All are available on the official PROMIS Web site (www.healthnetwork.net). Apps are available to administer these using a tablet computer (for a fee). Validated PROMIS measures completed on paper (eg, PROMIS 29, PROMIS 10) are best used for research purposes. Research and EHR systems are incorporating PROMIS CATs, short forms, or profiles into their software (**Table 4**). The CATs efficiently reduce the number items needed to assess each domain; 7 to 8 domains can be answered in 5 to 8 minutes. CATs implementation should be the goal for all PROMIS uses.

Table 4
Mechanisms to capture PROMIS outcomes electronically using computerized adaptive test systems (CATs)

Health Network	
Assessment center	Web-based data-collection platform
Assessment center application programming interface (API)	API connects data-collection software with all CATs and PROMIS measures
Electronic health record (EHR) systems	
Epic	EHR software: has selected PROMIS measures since 2012
Research-based systems	
REDCap	Web application for building and managing online surveys
OBERD	Enterprise software supports capture of PROMIS outcomes

TBD REF website and date accessed.

THE VALIDITY OF PATIENT-REPORTED OUTCOMES MEASUREMENT INFORMATION SYSTEM IN RHEUMATIC DISEASES

Multiple validation studies have been performed using PROMIS measures and short forms. A recent summary of multiple validation studies justifies the use of PROMIS measures or short forms across varied clinical populations, including

Table 5
Recent studies for validation of PROMIS in rheumatic diseases (2017–2018)

Reference, Year	Rheumatic Disease(s)	PROMIS Instruments for Validation	Validation Approach
Kasturi et al,[26] 2018	SLE	PROMIS 10-Global	Feasible, construct validity
Kasturi et al,[25] 2018	SLE	PROMIS CATs	Construct validity
Khanna et al,[27] 2017	SSc	PROMIS GI Measures	Responsiveness
Li et al,[28] 2018	RA	10-item PF	Low implementation with paper copies and in minorities
Kwakkenbos et al,[29] 2017	SSc	PROMIS29 V2.0	Construct validity, QoL
Wahl et al,[23] 2017	RA	10-Item PF SF	Construct validity and responsiveness
Katz et al,[30] 2017	RA, OA, FM, SLE	PROMIS29	Construct validity, floor-ceiling
Izadi et al,[31] 2018	RA	10-Item PF SF	Possible loss of reliability in people with non–English language proficiency
Wohlfahrt et al,[32] 2018	RA	8 PROMIS CATs	Responsiveness with intervention
Bartlett et al,[33] 2018	RA[a]	PROMIS SF	Content validity, language
Yost et al,[34] 2017	FM	PROMIS Fatigue	Construct validity

Abbreviations: CATs, computerized adaptive testing system; FM, fibromyalgia; GI, gastrointestinal; OA, osteoarthritis; PF, physical function; QoL, quality of life; RA, rheumatoid arthritis; SF, short form; SLE, systemic lupus erythematosus; SSc, systemic sclerosis.

[a] All studies evaluated patients in settings of usual care and one study tested subjects in an online database.

rheumatic and orthopedic conditions, supporting it use in clinical and comparative effectiveness research.[20,21] These include validation of reliability and construct validity of 11 PROMIS instruments in people with rheumatoid arthritis (RA) of RA-relevant selected PROMIS instruments.[22,23] Over the past 2 years, several studies have demonstrated the construct validity, feasibility, meaningful thresholds, and responsiveness of PROMIS measures in rheumatic diseases with complex clinical manifestations (**Table 5**). Research into relationships between PROMIS health states and complex phenotypes of rheumatic disease are ongoing.[24–26]

One study assessing PROMIS29 measures across 4 rheumatic diseases demonstrated domain scores varied from referent norms, as would be expected for each condition, with excellent internal consistency, supporting generalizability across rheumatic disease states.[30] The PROMIS 29 met criteria for validity in systemic sclerosis and demonstrated reduction in QoL due to gastrointestinal symptoms and hand contractures.[29] One group demonstrated that the change in the clinical disease activity (CDAI) index in patients with RA following intervention correlated with changes in PROMIS measures of physical health, pain, and sleep, suggesting a role for measuring these in settings of care and between visits when patients cannot always attend clinic visits.[32] Other studies demonstrated construct validity for PROMIS fatigue in patients with RA and fibromyalgia.[30,34,35]

IS THERE STILL A ROLE FOR USING LEGACY QUESTIONNAIRES?

The Rationale for Switching from Legacy Patient-Reported Outcomes to Patient-Reported Outcomes Measurement Information System

Unlike PROMIS measures and profiles, which were developed and validated using modern measurement science, including IRT, most Legacy PROs were developed using clinimetric methods and scored using CTT. This approach is less psychometrically sound. When administering PROMIS CATs, scores have higher precision/reduced error, reduced floor and ceiling effects, and interpretation is linked to the norm. Often the best Legacy PRO items have already been incorporated into PROMIS item banks, but now they can be applied across diseases. Thus, PROMIS measures can be used across multiple orthopedic and rheumatic conditions, using fewer items.

PROMIS measures were intended for use in BOTH research and care and can enhance communication between clinicians and patients in clinical settings.[34] They are available in multiple languages, so in settings of care they enhance patient-provider communication, can improve patient-centered choices and decision making, and can demonstrate value in care. The standardized system of health assessment with harmonized, calibrated scoring metrics makes PROMIS measures and profiles ideal for research when comparing safety and effectiveness of interventions, and data from multiple studies can be more easily meta-analyzed to establish high levels of evidence of interventions, and cost-effectiveness.

The question arises when PRO assessment can almost completely rely on the PROMIS system. Given the limitations in precision, reliability, and comparability among Legacy PROs, there is a need to move away from their use. This will require means to overcome any barriers to PROMIS implementation to maximize provider, patient, and researcher experience with PROMIS measures.

Cross-Walking Legacy Patient-Reported Outcomes to Patient-Reported Outcomes Measurement Information System

The accuracy of transforming (cross-walking) disease-specific Legacy PRO scores to PROMIS T-scores and vice versa remains a concern for researchers and others implementing PROs. Lapin and colleagues[37] assessed this by performing a study to examine precision of cross-walking of VR-RAND scores to PROMIS 10 Global Mental and Physical Health summary scores using previously published tables for 4606 patients seen in spine clinic from October 2015 to 2016. Their analyses of both scores showed high levels of agreement between VR-RAND and PROMIS-10 summary scores. They also used bootstrapping statistical techniques to demonstrate precision could be maintained for samples sizes as low as 200 patients, concluding that VR-12 and PROMIS Global Health scores can be accurately linked, and sample sizes of 200 patients could be used for comparative effectiveness studies.

Implementing Patient-Reported Outcomes Measurement Information System in Settings of Care

The utility of implementing PROMIS into practice is still being investigated. A recent qualitative indicated patients were cautiously enthusiastic of integrating symptom-based PROs (sleep, pain, anxiety, depression, and low energy [fatigue] or SPADE) that normally go unrecognized. Patient-endorsed completed PROs could foster communication and clinical action but not if PROs were too long, unvalued, nonprioritized, or unused. They concurred visual displays would be useful.[38] In a comprehensive review of 31 of 447 potential Legacy and Generic PROs considered as being feasible to systematically include in practice to facilitate patient-provider communication around hip and knee osteoarthritis (OA), PROMIS short forms assessing pain physical function, fatigue, and sleep were endorsed for being brief; enabling in-depth or detailed assessment; being of low burden to patients, providers, and staff; and relevant to OA management. Moreover, they were publicly accessible and had demonstrated validity and reliability in patients with OA.[39]

Rational for Using the Patient-Reported Outcomes Measurement Information System Computerized Adaptive Testing System in Clinical Settings

PROMIS CATs is the most efficient method for administering PROMIS measures. Probabilistic response-based algorithms, derived using IRT, limits response burden and time. Patient-calibrated scores can be determined for each 7 to 8 core domains in less than 10 minutes[40] in a range of clinical settings. If regularly completed before clinical encounters, scores could provide insights into new health problems, trigger a more targeted and relevant discussion between provider and patient, and lead to higher quality of care.

Patient-Reported Outcomes Measurement Information System Computerized Adaptive Testing System in Clinical Care

The ability to rapidly self-assess multiple health domains enriches information available to providers and can, in turn, enhance patient-centered care with the potential to improve the quality and satisfaction of care, adherence to therapy, and address factors such as social participation more efficiently than in traditional EHR-burdened patient encounters. In a study of 280 patients with RA completing PROMIS CATs for 8 RA-relevant core domains, both patients and their providers found the CATs visual graphs of domain scores relative to the norm useful, increasing awareness and communication around health issues, and improving the quality of the clinical encounter[36]

The implementation of PROMIS in settings of care has been inconsistent. Despite evidence of construct validity, responsiveness, and feasibility of the PROMIS CATs, they cannot be useful in care unless they are integrated into EHRs. A recent study demonstrated a 15% increase in completion of PROMIS function short forms when completed digitally versus on paper, but white English-speaking individuals were more likely to do so compared with minority patients.[31] Further efforts are needed to understand how PROMIS will be received, particularly among differing race/ethnic groups.[28] Most providers are unaware of the PROMIS and evidence is lacking to demonstrate practical value in settings of care.

Even the PROMIS 10, which is easy to administer, requires standardized procedures to be in place to ensure patients complete these before each clinical encounter. Easy access to CATs completion and graphical interfaces that readily display scores and reference norms could enable providers and patients to view them together. Doctors could have a greater understanding of each patient's experience with his or her health, leading to more relevant, focused, and meaningful clinical interchange and more informed treatment decisions.[36] If PROs become part of meaningful use, administrators would facilitate integration of patients' assessments into clinical care pathways and into EHRs. However, further study is needed to assess whether lower health literacy and non-English speakers might require the use of pictograms when administering items to overcome health literacy issues. Providers need to understand PROMIS measures relative to the Legacy questionnaires they are using in practice settings when monitoring treatment responses, side effects, or making treatment decisions for specific diseases. Although digital Apps are becoming available, they are still costly. Some practice environments prefer to use only value-based profiles to assess health utilities and quality of care, thus use of the PROMIS 10 global is the profile of choice. This is being examined in patients with systemic lupus erythematosus examining patient preferences and feasibility of using short forms and CATs in the clinic.[26]

FUTURE USE OF PATIENT-REPORTED OUTCOMES MEASUREMENT INFORMATION SYSTEM MEASURES AND SHORT FORMS IN ECOLOGICAL MONITORING USING SMART PHONES

Reports are emerging demonstrating the use of PROMIS measures and data using smart phone applications for interventional n of 1 trials and as part of a multidimensional assessments that incorporate novel PROs and image-based measures.[41,42] As PROMIS measures become integrated into EHR systems linked to patient portals and more smart phone applications, it is conceivable that PROMIS-based self-assessments will become standard in patient assessments improving the quality of patient-provider encounters and care. Currently a smart phone application is available from the PROMIS Web site for a fee.

SUMMARY

PROMIS is a tool to elicit self-reported health status that can be presented using a T-score metric, standardized and calibrated to compare scores of health status domains relative to the normal population. Questions are geared to adults and reflect a continuum of possible response options from very low ability or severe symptoms or impact to high ability or absence of symptoms or impact. It has now been validated across many illnesses, conditions, and procedures. PROMIS measures accurately and reliably estimate the health status of key core domains and can be applied to many disorders and procedures. PROMIS measures have been validated for health assessment, prediction of response to treatment, assessment of treatment responses, and can be feasibly integrated into practice, and even between clinical encounters. To transition to only the use of PROMIS will take time, as researchers and clinicians still need additional information to be convinced of their utility and meaningfulness. Exchanging Legacy PROs for PROMIS is a big leap, as interpretation of the measures is not fully elucidated. Each institution will need to determine which measures, short forms, or profiles should be included. If incorporated into their EHR, people will need to ensure it is immediately scored and standardized scores are provided right away.

REFERENCES

1. Cella D, Riley W, Stone A, et al. The patient-reported outcomes measurement information system (PROMIS) developed and tested its first wave of adult selfreported health outcome item banks: 2005-2008. J Clin Epidemiol 2010;63(11): 1179–94.
2. Lillegraven S, Kvien TK. Measuring disability and quality of life in established rheumatoid arthritis. Best Pract Res Clin Rheumatol 2007;21(5):827–40.
3. Bykerk VP, Bingham CO, Choy EH, et al. Identifying flares in rheumatoid arthritis: reliability and construct validation of the OMERACT RA Flare Core Domain Set. RMD Open 2016;2(1):e000225.14.
4. Pincus T, Swearingen CJ, Bergman M, et al. RAPID 3 (routine assessment of patient index data 3), a rheumatoid arthritis index without formal joint counts for routine care: proposed severity categories compared to disease activity score and clinical disease activity index categories. J Rheumatol 2008;35(11):2136–47.
5. D C. Available at: http://www.healthmeasures.net/explore-measurement-systems/promis/intro-to-promis. Accessed February 20, 2019.
6. Available at: https://www.aci.health.nsw.gov.au/__data/assets/pdf_file/0003/402087/ Overview-of-the-PROMIS-29_EH-140817.pdf. Accessed November 27, 2018.
7. De Vet HCW, Terwee CB, Mokkink LB, et al. Measurement in medicine: a practical guide (practical guides to biostatistics and epidemiology). 1st edition. Cambridge (United Kingdom): Cambridge University Press; 2011.
8. Pilkonis PA, Choi SW, Reise SP, et al, PROMIS Cooperative Group. Item banks for measuring emotional distress from the Patient-Reported Outcomes Measurement Information System (PROMIS): depression, anxiety, and anger. Assessment 2011;18(3):263–83.
9. Available at: http://www.healthmeasures.net/explore-measurement-systems/promis. Accessed February 19, 2019.
10. Available at: http://www.healthmeasures.net/explore-measurement-systems/promis/intro-to-promis/list-of-adult-measures. Accessed February 20, 2019.
11. Revicki DA, Kawata AK, Harnam N, et al. Predicting EuroQol (EQ-5D) scores from the patient-reported outcomes measurement information system (PROMIS) global items and domain item banks in a United States sample. Qual Life Res 2009;18(6):783–91.
12. Cella D, Riley W, Stone A, et al. The Patient-Reported Outcomes Measurement Information System (PROMIS) developed and tested its first wave of adult self-reported health outcome item banks: 2005±2008. J Clin Epidemiol 2010;63(11): 1179–94.
13. Hanmer J, Cella D, Feeny D, et al. Selection of key health domains from PROMIS for a generic preference-based scoring system. Qual Life Res 2017;26(12): 3377–85.
14. Hanmer J, Dewitt B, Yu L, et al. Cross-sectional validation of the PROMIS-Preference scoring system. PLoS One 2018;13(7):e0201093.

15. Thompson NR, Lapin BR, Katzan IL. Mapping PROMIS global health items to EuroQol (EQ-5D) utility scores using linear and equipercentile equating. Pharmacoeconomics 2017;35(11):1167–76.
16. Nguyen TH, Han HR, Kim MT, et al. An introduction to item response theory for patient-reported outcome measurement. Patient 2014;7(1):23–35.
17. Choi SW, Schalet B, Cook KF, et al. Establishing a common metric for depressive symptoms: linking the BDI-II, CES-D, and PHQ-9 to PROMIS depression. Psychol Assess 2014;26(2):513–27.
18. Fries JF, Witter J, Rose M, et al. Item response theory, computerized adaptive testing, and PROMIS: assessment of physical function. J Rheumatol 2014;41(1):153–8.
19. Bingham CO 3rd, Bartlett SJ, Merkel PA, et al. Using patient-reported outcomes and PROMIS in research and clinical applications: experiences from the PCORI pilot projects. Qual Life Res 2016;25(8):2109–16.
20. Cook KF, Jensen SE, Schalet BD, et al. PROMIS measures of pain, fatigue, negative affect, physical function, and social function demonstrated clinical validity across a range of chronic conditions. J Clin Epidemiol 2016;73:89–102.
21. Beleckas CM, Padovano A, Guattery J, et al. Performance of patient-reported outcomes measurement information system (PROMIS) upper extremity (UE) versus physical function (PF) computer adaptive tests (CATs) in upper extremity clinics. J Hand Surg 2017;42(11):867–74.
22. Bartlett SJ, Hewlett S, Bingham CO 3rd, et al. Identifying core domains to assess flare in rheumatoid arthritis: an OMERACT international patient and provider combined Delphi consensus. Ann Rheum Dis 2012;71(11):1855–60.
23. Wahl E, Gross A, Chernitskiy V, et al. Validity and responsiveness of a 10-item patient-reported measure of physical function in a rheumatoid arthritis clinic population. Arthritis Care Res 2017;69(3):338–46.
24. Kasturi S, Burket JC, Berman JR, et al. Feasibility of Patient-Reported Outcomes Measurement Information System (PROMIS(R)) computerized adaptive tests in systemic lupus erythematosus outpatients. Lupus 2018;27(10):1591–9.
25. Kasturi S, Szymonifka J, Burket JC, et al. Validity and reliability of patient reported outcomes measurement information system computerized adaptive tests in systemic lupus erythematosus. J Rheumatol 2017;44(7):1024–31.
26. Kasturi S, Szymonifka J, Burket JC, et al. Feasibility, validity, and reliability of the 10-item patient reported outcomes measurement information system global health short form in outpatients with systemic lupus erythematosus. J Rheumatol 2018;45(3):397–404.
27. Khanna D, Serrano J, Berrocal VJ, et al. A randomized controlled trial to evaluate an Internet-based self-management program in systemic sclerosis. Arthritis Care Res (Hoboken) 2018. [Epub ahead of print].
28. Li J, Yazdany J, Trupin L, et al. Capturing a patient-reported measure of physical function through an online electronic health record patient portal in an ambulatory clinic: implementation study. JMIR Med Inform 2018;6(2):e31.
29. Kwakkenbos L, Thombs BD, Khanna D, et al. Performance of the patient-reported outcomes measurement information system-29 in scleroderma: a scleroderma patient-centered intervention network cohort study. Rheumatology (Oxford) 2017;56(8):1302–11.
30. Katz P, Pedro S, Michaud K. Performance of the patient-reported outcomes measurement information system 29-item profile in rheumatoid arthritis, osteoarthritis, fibromyalgia, and systemic lupus erythematosus. Arthritis Care Res 2017;69(9):1312–21.

31. Izadi Z, Katz PP, Schmajuk G, et al. Effects of language, insurance and race/ethnicity on measurement properties of the PROMIS Physical Function Short Form 10a in rheumatoid arthritis. Arthritis Care Res (Hoboken) 2018. [Epub ahead of print].
32. Wohlfahrt A, Bingham CO 3rd, Marder W, et al. Responsiveness of patient reported outcomes measurement information system (PROMIS) measures in RA patients starting or switching a DMARD. Arthritis Care Res (Hoboken) 2018. [Epub ahead of print].
33. Bartlett SJ, Witter J, Cella D, et al. Montreal accord on patient-reported outcomes (PROs) use series - paper 6: creating national initiatives to support development and use-the PROMIS example. J Clin Epidemiol 2017;89:148–53.
34. Yost KJ, Waller NG, Lee MK, et al. The PROMIS fatigue item bank has good measurement properties in patients with fibromyalgia and severe fatigue. Qual Life Res 2017;26(6):1417–26.
35. Bartlett SJ, Gutierrez AK, Butanis A, et al. Combining online and in-person methods to evaluate the content validity of PROMIS fatigue short forms in rheumatoid arthritis. Qual Life Res 2018;27(9):2443–51.
36. Bingham C III. Making PROMIS meaningful to patients and providers in clinical practice. Available at: https://www.pcori.org/research-results/2014/making-promismeaningful-patients-and-providers-clinical-practice. Accessed November 29, 2018.
37. Lapin BR, Kinzy TG, Thompson NR, et al. Accuracy of linking VR-12 and PROMIS global health scores in clinical practice. Value in health 2018;21(10):1226–33.
38. Talib TL, DeChant P, Kean J, et al. A qualitative study of patients' perceptions of the utility of patient-reported outcome measures of symptoms in primary care clinics. Qual Life Res 2018;27(12):3157–66.
39. Golightly YM, Allen KD, Nyrop KA, et al. Patient-reported outcomes to initiate a provider-patient dialog for the management of hip and knee osteoarthritis. Semin Arthritis Rheum 2015;42(2):123–31.
40. Schifferdecker KE, Yount SE, Kaiser K, et al. A method to create a standardized generic and condition-specific patient-reported outcome measure for patient care and healthcare improvement. Qual Life Res 2018;27(2):367–78.
41. Kravitz RL, Schmid CH, Marois M, et al. Effect of mobile device-supported single-patient multi-crossover trials on treatment of chronic musculoskeletal pain: a randomized clinical trial. JAMA Intern Med 2018;178(10):1368–77.
42. Mollard E, Michaud K. A mobile app with optical imaging for the selfmanagement of hand rheumatoid arthritis: pilot study. JMIR MHealth UHealth 2018;6(10):e12221.

Motivational Counseling and Text Message Reminders

For Reduction of Daily Sitting Time and Promotion of Everyday Physical Activity in People with Rheumatoid Arthritis

Tanja Thomsen, OT, MScH, PhD[a,*],
Bente Appel Esbensen, RN, MSciN, PhD[a,b],
Merete Lund Hetland, MD, PhD, DMSc[a,b,c],
Mette Aadahl, PT, MPH, PhD[d,e]

KEYWORDS

• Sedentary behavior • Physical activity • Rheumatoid arthritis
• Behavioral interventions • Motivational counseling • Text message reminders

KEY POINTS

- Patients with rheumatoid arthritis tend to be physically inactive and sedentary.
- Physical inactivity and sedentary behavior are associated with an increased risk of cardiovascular disease in patients with rheumatoid arthritis.
- Reduction of daily sitting time replaced by light-intensity physical activity emerges as a simple and suitable approach to generate health-related benefits and long-term compliance in patients with rheumatoid arthritis.
- Individual behavioral interventions supported by technology are promising facilitators in promoting physical activity and reducing sedentary behavior in patients with rheumatoid arthritis.

Disclosure Statement: The authors have no conflicts of interest or disclosures to declare in relation to this article.

[a] Copenhagen Center for Arthritis Research, Center for Rheumatology and Spine Diseases, Centre for Head and Orthopaedics, Rigshospitalet, Nordre Ringvej 57, Indgang 5, Glostrup, DK-2600, Denmark; [b] Department of Clinical Medicine, Faculty of Health and Medical Sciences, University of Copenhagen, Copenhagen, Denmark; [c] The DANBIO Registry, Center for Rheumatology and Spine Diseases, Centre for Head and Orthopaedics, Rigshospitalet, Nordre Ringvej 57, Indgang 5, Glostrup, DK-2600, Denmark; [d] Centre for Clinical Research and Prevention, Bispebjerg and Frederiksberg Hospital, Nordre Fasanvej 57, Hovedvejen 5, Frederiksberg 2000, Denmark; [e] Department of Public Health, Faculty of Health and Medical Sciences, University of Copenhagen, Blegdamsvej 3B, 2200 Copenhagen N, Denmark
* Corresponding author.
E-mail address: tanja.thomsen@regionh.dk

Rheum Dis Clin N Am 45 (2019) 231–244
https://doi.org/10.1016/j.rdc.2019.01.005
0889-857X/19/

INTRODUCTION

For more than a decade, there has been a growing interest in strategies to increase participation in physical activity in people with rheumatoid arthritis (RA).[1,2] The large number of intervention studies includes both cardiorespiratory aerobic exercise and resistance exercise training,[1,2] and there is good evidence that moderate and vigorous physical activity (MVPA) has a positive impact on cardiovascular health, disease-related symptoms, and physical function in RA.[2,3] However, there is limited evidence that MVPA is increased and maintained on a long-term basis in patients with RA. A suggested alternative approach is reducing sedentary behavior and replacing it with light-intensity physical activity, which may serve as a gateway to higher levels of physical activity in patients with RA.[4,5]

Defining Physical Activity, Physical Inactivity, and Sedentary Behavior

In this regard, it is important to recognize the definitions of physical activity, physical inactivity, and sedentary behavior. Physical activity refers to any bodily movement generated by skeletal muscle that results in energy expenditure.[6] Physical inactivity refers to not meeting general recommendations of MVPA,[6] and although no formal consensus has been reached, sedentary behavior has been defined as "*Any waking behavior characterized by an energy expenditure less than or equal to 1.5 metabolic equivalent of task (MET) while in a sitting or reclining position*,"[7] that is, corresponding to the low end of the so-called continuum of physical activity energy expenditure (**Fig. 1**). Sedentary behavior comprises behaviors such as desk work, reading, motorized transportation, television viewing, or other screen-based activities.[8]

Physical Activity Recommendations for Patients with Rheumatoid Arthritis

Patients with RA, as well as the general population, are recommended to meet general physical activity guidelines, that is, participate in moderate physical activity for at least 150 minutes per week.[9] Specifically, patients with RA are recommended to engage in aerobic exercise and resistance training, supervised initially and tailored to the patient's disease activity and disease manifestations.[10] These recommendations are supported by a recent literature review and meta-analysis from the European League Against Rheumatism (EULAR).[11] The meta-analysis resulted in a range of physical activity recommendations for patients with osteoarthritis (OA), RA, and spondyloarthritis.[11] An overarching principle was that physical activity should be viewed as a general concept to optimize health-related quality of life (QoL) in patients with inflammatory arthritis (IA) and OA. As such, it was recommended that promoting physical activity consistent with general physical activity recommendations should be an integral part of standard care throughout the course of disease in patients with these

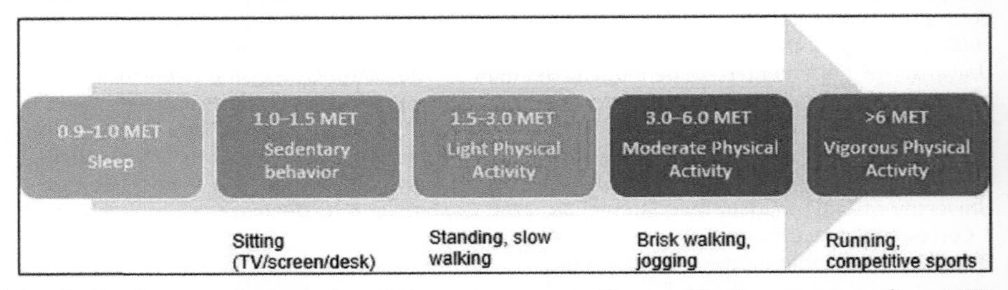

Fig. 1. Continuum of physical activity energy expenditure with the corresponding METs. (*Adapted from* Overgaard K, Grontved A, Nielsen K, et al. Stillesiddende adfærd—en helbredsrisiko? 1st edition. Copenhagen (Denmark): Vidensraad for Forebyggelse; 2012.)

diagnoses. Recommending physical activity as part of the treatment will also require a shared decision between health care providers and the patients, which takes patients' preferences, capabilities, and resources into account and addresses general and disease-specific barriers and facilitators related to performing physical activity, including knowledge, social support, and symptom control.[11]

Current Strategies to Promote Physical Activity in Patients with Rheumatoid Arthritis

Several studies have explored interventions that aim to optimize physical activity in patients with RA.[2,12,13] These interventions can be broadly grouped into those using aerobic exercise training and/or muscle strengthening training and those applying behavioral approaches, for example, counseling and goal setting. Supervised exercise programs allow a regular and direct interaction with health professionals with an immediate possibility to relieve potential RA symptoms and initiate changes in physical activity behavior. Documentation for whether these exercise programs alone can increase physical activity in patients with RA is limited.[1,12] Behavioral approaches often involve specific behavior change techniques with or without a theoretic basis.[13] Both types of interventions, that is, those involving exercise programs and those including behavioral approaches, have shown varying results with respect to promoting physical activity behavior in patients with RA.[2,13] Still, the EULAR physical activity recommendations[11] highlight that health care providers should deliver physical activity interventions that include self-monitoring, goal setting, action planning, feedback, and problem solving.[11] The literature has called for further studies that seek to develop and implement the optimal intervention to change behavior in the RA population.[12,13]

Physical Activity and Sedentary Behavior in Patients with Rheumatoid Arthritis

It is well established that there are several health benefits of engaging in MVPA for patients with RA; it appears to be safe for the joints and improves QoL and important RA-related outcomes, such as pain and physical function.[1] However, patients with RA have reported multiple barriers to engaging in regular exercise and performing usual leisure-time activities, including pain, fatigue, decreased physical function,[14] fear of damaging the joints, and lack of motivation and knowledge.[12] In addition, the literature indicates that health professionals also lack knowledge of how to promote and provide guidance on physical activity in patients with RA.[12,15] Therefore, this is not undertaken consistently in clinical practice.[15] These barriers are probably reflected in cross-sectional data (N = 5235), suggesting that up to 60% to 80% of patients with RA have not adopted recommendations of MVPA and exercise,[16] and that most patients with RA spend on average only 0.2 h/d in MVPA.[17,18] In addition, there is increasing evidence that patients with RA spend a larger proportion of their waking hours in sedentary behaviors compared with the general population,[17–19] that is, 90% to 95% versus 60% to 70% of waking hours[19,20] (**Fig. 2**).

The main reported reasons for sedentary behavior and prolonged sitting in everyday lives of patients with RA comprise RA-related symptoms (fatigue, pain, decreased physical function) and a strategy chosen in order to cope with the fluctuating nature of the disease through the planning of frequent periods with rest and sitting time.[21]

Sedentary Behavior and Health-Related Outcomes

Sedentary behavior and its associations with health-related outcomes have become a rapidly increasing research area, and a substantial amount of scientific

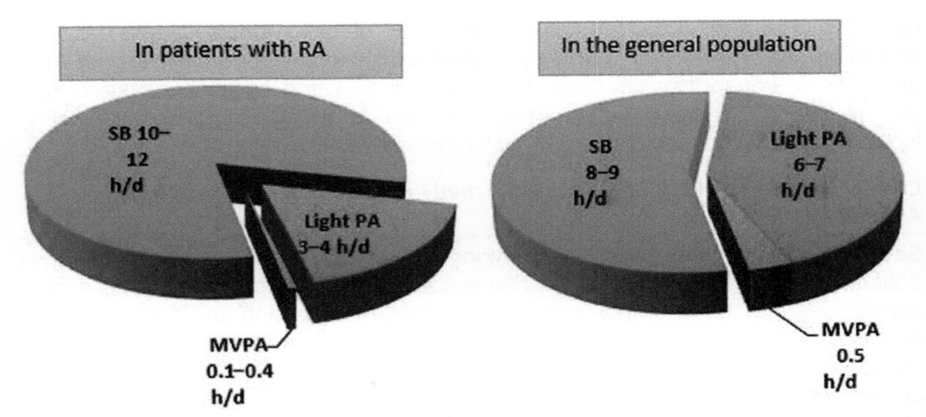

Fig. 2. Physical activity levels during 16 waking hours. PA, physical activity; SB, sedentary behavior. (*Data from* Refs.[17,19,49,50])

literature on sedentary behavior in adults has been accumulated.[22,23] There is now a consistent base of epidemiologic evidence reporting associations of sedentary behavior with increased risk of type 2 diabetes, cardiovascular disease, overweight and obesity, and all-cause mortality.[22–24] Noticeably, the adverse health outcomes of prolonged sitting have also been found in people who report at least 2.5 hours of weekly MVPA,[25] although the greatest health risk exists in those individuals who are both physically inactive and sedentary.[26] Accordingly, a recent meta-analysis has indicated that an individual needs to engage in 60 to 75 minutes of daily MVPA to eliminate the increased risk of all-cause mortality associated with high sitting time.[26] Because RA itself is associated with an increased risk of cardiovascular disease, an everyday life without meeting MVPA recommendations combined with prolonged sitting may further elevate this risk.[27] This risk calls for an increased awareness of promoting physical activity in patients with RA.

Replacing Sedentary Behavior with Light Physical Activity

Based on cross-sectional data documenting that sedentary behavior and light-intensity physical activity are strongly inversely associated,[28] it may be assumed that individuals engage more in standing and stepping activities when reducing time spent in sedentary behaviors. The relatively new health promotion approach of reducing sedentary behavior and replacing it with light-intensity physical activity has been tested in a variety of settings and populations of healthy adults with positive results in terms of reduced total daily sitting time,[29] television viewing,[30] and occupational sitting,[31,32] and with improvements in fasting serum insulin levels,[29] waist circumference,[29] high-density lipoprotein cholesterol,[32] and energy expenditure.[30] Based on these promising results, a similar approach has been suggested for groups of patients with chronic disease and functional limitations. Accordingly, and not disregarding the important health benefits of engaging in MVPA and exercise, earlier research has advocated reduction of sedentary behavior to be replaced by light-intensity physical activity as a potentially more feasible and achievable health promotion strategy for patients with chronic disease and/or mobility limitations.[4] However, there is very limited evidence on if and how it is possible to reduce sedentary behavior in these populations.

An Example of an Intervention Aiming to Reduce Sedentary Behavior in Patients with Rheumatoid Arthritis

As the first study to focus on sedentary behavior replaced by light-intensity physical activity in patients with RA, a randomized controlled trial (N = 150), the Joint Resources–Sedentary Behavior (JR-SB) study,[33,34] was recently conducted. The trial aimed to investigate the efficacy of an individually tailored, behavioral intervention on objectively measured daily sitting time, clinical patient-reported outcomes, and cardiometabolic biomarkers. Participants were invited to the study through screening of eligibility via the DANBIO database.[35]

The 4-month intervention had a theoretic basis with emphasis on behavioral choice theory,[36] which describes how individuals replace the choice of an unhealthy behavior with a healthier alternative, for example, replacing a night of television watching with an evening walk. In addition, the theoretic framework included the concept of self-efficacy as described by Bandura,[37] that is, the participant's belief in his/her own skills to reduce sedentary behavior. Furthermore, it incorporated behavior change and motivational interviewing techniques.[38] More specifically, the intervention consisted of (1) Three individual motivational counseling sessions, conducted by a health professional (registered nurse or occupational therapist); (2) Four key messages; and (3) Individual daily/weekly text message reminders, which the participants received between the 3 counseling sessions.

Motivational counseling

In the first motivational counseling session, the participant was encouraged to identify daily patterns of sedentary behavior, and at the same time, current scientific knowledge of sedentary behavior and adverse health outcomes were discussed between the participant and the interviewer. The session also incorporated individual behavioral goal setting and action planning for change in sedentary behavior in a domain after his/her own choice (at work, during leisure time, and/or motorized transportation).[33] In the 2 subsequent counseling sessions, behavioral goals were reviewed, including a dialogue between participant and interviewer about pros and cons of the outcomes of the behavior, identity associated with the changed behavior, and feedback on the behavior from the interviewer. Accordingly, the behavioral goals were modified or new ones were set.[33] **Fig. 3** provides an overview of the intervention.

Four key messages

During the 3 counseling sessions, the participants were provided with 4 booklets, each containing a key message related to reduction of sedentary behavior, and with specific suggestions to reduce and break up daily sitting time. These key messages focused on the following: (1) Reduction of TV viewing; (2) Substitution of sitting with standing when possible, at work and at home; (3) Breaks in prolonged sitting by standing up frequently; and (4) A maximum of 30 minutes of sitting per episode.[33]

Text message reminders

Immediately after each motivational counseling session, an external communications consultant drafted individually tailored text messages to the participant reminding him/her of his/her own behavioral goals of reducing daily sitting time. In order to tailor the messages as specific as possible, it was an important intervention feature that the communications consultant was provided with the individual participant's personal data, including age, sex, partner status, housing (eg, whether the participant lived in an apartment, townhouse, single family house, and so forth) and leisure-time activities. This registration of personal data was done to avoid "unrealistic" reminders sent to the participants, for example, by asking a single woman to take along her partner on the

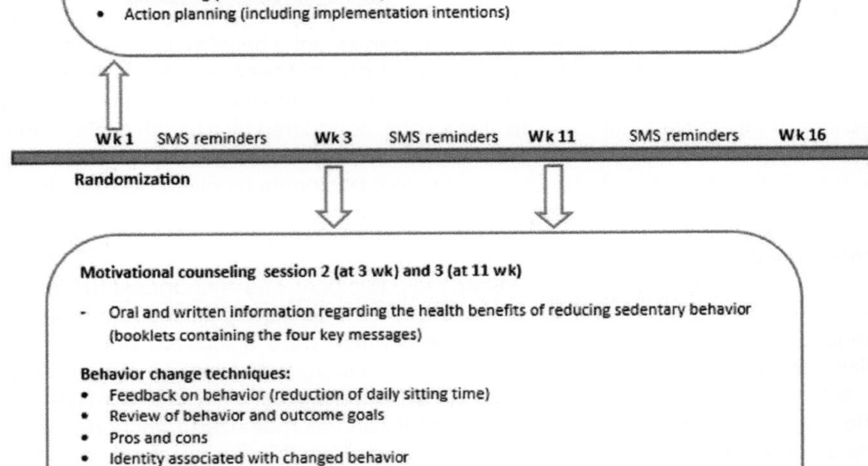

Fig. 3. A time schedule of the intervention and the applied behavior change techniques. (*From* Thomsen T, Aadahl M, Beyer N, et al. Motivational counselling and SMS-reminders for reduction of daily sitting time in patients with rheumatoid arthritis: a descriptive randomised controlled feasibility study. BMC Musculoskelet Disord 2016;17(1):434; with permission.)

evening walk or encourage a man without a garden to reduce his TV watching and replace it with garden work. The participants decided the frequency and timing of the messages with a maximum of 5 messages per week for each participant. SMS-tracking Apps (https://www.smstrack.com/) developed and monitored the technical system, supporting the sending of the text messages. **Table 1** shows examples of behavioral goals and the corresponding SMS reminders from a preconducted feasibility study.[33]

At short-term follow-up, immediately after the 4-month intervention period, patients in the intervention group had reduced their daily sitting time by on average 1.6 h/d (assessed objectively by an ActivPAL monitor) compared with an increase

Table 1
Examples of behavioral goals and the corresponding text message reminders based on the 4 key messages

Individual Goals of Reducing Daily Sitting Time	Actual SMS Reminder
Reduction of daily TV viewing	Hi X. If commercials are on why not go and get a refreshing glass of water? Hi X. Start your laundry before you sit down to watch TV and give it a check next time there are commercials. Maybe it needs drying or folding. Hi X. Give your body a good stretch and why not do the dishes while you wait for the commercials to finish? Hi X. Have you been sitting for long in front of the TV today? If you take your old newspapers down to the container, then you recycle and get a mouthful of fresh air at the same time.
Substitution of sitting with standing when possible: at work, at home, or during transportation	Hi X. This morning, on your way to work, why not stand up in the aisle for the last 2 stops before you get off the train? Hi X. Let gravity assist in digesting your lunch; raise your table and work standing up the next hour. You might even inspire your colleagues. Hi X. Are you on your way home from work? If the sun is shining, why not get off the bus a stop earlier than usual? Remember to enjoy the weather while you walk. Hi X. Next time the phone rings, why not hold the conversation standing up? Walking alone is great, but better together. Take your husband by the hand, and enjoy the warm and bright evening.
Break up prolonged sitting: by standing up frequently	Hi X. Are you doing your crosswords? For every sixth word you do, get up and get yourself a glass of water or a piece of fruit. Hi X. Anything interesting in the newspaper today? When you finish the next article, get up and stretch your legs and maybe put another log on the fire.
Maximum 30 min of sitting per episode	Hi X. Before you sit down at your computer this afternoon, start a project that needs your attention once in a while. Maybe your laundry if you have booked the machines. Hi X. If the weather allows it, put your sewing away and take a swing down by the lake. There might be some hungry ducks if you bring some bread. Hi X. At tonight's poker game you can be the one getting drinks for the others, for example, every time cards are dealt. It would surely be appreciated. Hi X. It is difficult to really appreciate the spring in the garden from a fourth-floor apartment. An activity for the coffee club today could be to go down and see the blooming plants and trees.

From Thomsen T, Aadahl M, Beyer N, et al. Motivational counselling and SMS-reminders for reduction of daily sitting time in patients with rheumatoid arthritis: a descriptive randomised controlled feasibility study. BMC Musculoskelet Disord 2016;17(1):434.

in the control group by 0.6 h/d. In the intervention group, 52 (70%) patients reduced their daily sitting time by at least 50 minutes compared with10 (14%) in the control group. In addition, the intervention patients reduced cholesterol levels and improved pain and fatigue compared with the usual lifestyle control group.[34] At the long-term follow-up, 22 months from baseline, the intervention group had maintained the reduction in daily sitting time by on average 1.1 h/d compared with an increase in controls by 1.32 h/d. The intervention patients had also maintained reductions in cholesterol levels, with additional reductions in levels of triglycerides and HbA_{1c}, compared with the control group. The improvements in patient-reported outcomes were also sustained.[39]

DISCUSSION

The associations of sedentary behavior with health outcomes and methods to reduce total daily sitting time and prolonged sitting in patients with RA are important areas for future research. There is still very limited evidence of effective strategies for reducing time spent in sedentary behaviors in this group of patients. However, the promising results from the JR-SB study underpin the use of behavioral approaches, that is, motivational counseling, information on health benefits, goal setting, and feedback on behavior from a health professional, to support the change of physical activity patterns in RA. These strategies are supported by the positive long-term results in the JR-SB study. Nevertheless, changing behavior is challenging, and behavioral interventions aimed at increasing physical activity in this context have had varying levels of success in patients with RA.[13] Another aspect, which may blur the picture regarding clear recommendations of how to reduce sedentary behavior/increase light-intensity physical in RA, is that behavioral interventions often use a combination of methods or behavior change techniques, making it difficult to conclude how well each of the intervention components contribute causally to the outcomes. The JR-SB study included written material, motivational interviewing, and specific behavior change techniques followed up by a technology element, that is, the individual SMS reminders, offered to the participants as a single package.[33,34] As such, it is unknown whether the motivational counseling sessions alone would have produced similar beneficial effects on the health outcomes. The literature advocates for further refinements of behavioral interventions targeting physical activity in patients with RA.[13,40]

Targeting Sedentary Behavior in Rheumatoid Arthritis in the Future: Elements to Consider

Reducing sedentary behavior is a new approach aiming to promote an overall more physically active lifestyle in everyday lives of patients with RA. Thus, apart from results from a single randomized controlled trial (JR-SB),[34] knowledge is lacking regarding effective behavioral strategies to reduce sedentary behavior in patients with RA. To plan and conduct future research in this regard, and for potential implementation in clinical practice, researchers may need to consider elements from physical activity interventions in patients with RA that have proven successful and draw on experiences from sedentary behavior interventions in other populations.

Identifying the targeted behavior

It seems that an important first step is being specific about the targeted behavior. A recent systematic review, including 51 randomized controlled trials in adult populations, concluded that interventions that targeted sedentary behavior alone were effective in reducing time spent sitting compared with interventions targeting physical activity alone or physical activity in conjunction with sedentary behavior.[41] This focus on sedentary behavior alone may automatically serve to increase physical activity because recent cross-sectional data have shown that right after time spent in sedentary behaviors, patients with RA spent most of their time in activities of very light or light intensity.[42] This replacing of behaviors was also reflected in the JR-SB study results because the reduced daily sitting time was mostly replaced by increased standing time, and to a lesser degree, by stepping time[34,39]

Motivational interviewing and coaching

Motivational interviewing is a counseling technique for encouraging people to make behavioral changes to improve health outcomes, which uses a broad range of communications skills.[38] These skills include open-ended questions, reflective listening, affirmation, and summarization in order to make individuals express thoughts, motivations, and concerns about change.[38] The method has been implemented in a variety of long-term conditions, addressing lifestyle changes with beneficial effects, but it is yet to be widely recognized and adopted in the field of rheumatology. Motivational interviewing was a key element in the JR-SB study and was found promising in order to reduce daily sitting time in patients with RA.[33]

However, the effect size of the counseling style is varied when it comes to promoting MVPA in RA populations. A recently conducted randomized controlled trial[40] evaluating the effect of a motivational interviewing-based lifestyle physical activity intervention on self-reported physical function in adults with knee OA or RA found no effect of the intervention for the RA participants.[40] The intervention consisted of 4 motivational counseling sessions during 12 months and focused on facilitating individualized lifestyle physical activity goal setting.[40] On the other hand, evidence has also suggested advantages in combining motivational interviewing with other behavioral approaches. Knittle and colleagues[43] documented that a motivational interview in conjunction with a group-based patient education session (both led by a physiotherapist) and 2 individual self-regulation coaching sessions (led by a nurse) proved effective in increasing leisure-time physical activity, number of active days per week, self-efficacy, and autonomous motivation (cognitions that predict physical activity initiation and maintenance). At both posttreatment (after 5 weeks) and 6-month follow-up, significantly more treated patients than controls met current physical activity recommendations.[43] In a later process evaluation, Knittle and colleagues[44] further argue that in promoting physical activity among patients with RA, supporting patient autonomy and teaching self-regulation skills, which focus attention on achieving physical activity goals, may improve long-term maintenance of physical activity.[44]

Use of technologies

New avenues to deliver interventions targeting physical activity and sedentary behavior are evolving rapidly, and an increasing number of researchers use modern technology and mobile health approaches to deliver physical activity–related interventions. A systematic review, published in 2018,[45] compiled evidence from randomized controlled trials (N = 5) evaluating the effectiveness of interactive digital interventions for physical activity and health-related QoL in patients with RA or juvenile idiopathic arthritis. The interventions should involve any digital platform (eg, computers, smart phones, or handheld devices, Web-based programs or applications) that underpinned a self-management component and included an interactive element. For instance, this could include activity logs, goal setting, discussion forums, task reminders, or physical activity monitoring. The results of the review indicated that there is limited evidence for the effect of interactive digital interventions on objectively measured physical activity in patients with RA immediately after the intervention or at least 1 year forward.[45]

However, none of the included interventions in the review used text messages to promote physical activity in the RA populations,[45] an intervention element that, based on the high frequency of optional text message reminders sent per week, was well received among the participants in the JR-SB study.[34] Although the use of text messages is recognized in health promotion interventions facilitating physical activity among older adults[46] and reduces sitting time in overweight/obese adults,[47] this method is not used to the same degree within rheumatology. Despite that, in a long-term follow-up of an intervention targeting promotion of health-enhancing physical activity in patients with RA (N = 177), Nordgren and colleagues[48] documented that in about one-fourth of originally sedentary individuals with RA, their new physical activity behaviors were sustained after 2 years. The multicomponent intervention included circuit training, support group meetings (including goal setting), and educational material about health-enhancing physical activity. The participants had free access to a Web page for registration and monitoring of their physical activity levels, and they were provided with weekly text messages to encourage their physical activity engagement.[48] The prompts from text messages together with coaching from health professionals were described as the most useful facilitators.[48]

Hence, although it appears feasible to use modern technology to deliver physical activity/sedentary behavior interventions targeting patients with RA, the inconclusive evidence emphasizes that the full potential of technology and mobile health in rheumatology has yet to be actualized. Data regarding specific features, delivery mode, and user preferences for content will potentially aid researchers in developing sedentary interventions that are relevant from the outset.

An individually tailored approach

For an effective intervention, it also seems important to acknowledge individual preferences, capabilities, and needs when targeting changes in physical activity and sedentary behavior in patients with RA.[34,43,48] Despite sufficient medical treatment of RA, patients still experience fluctuating levels of pain, fatigue, and physical function[21] and may need different or varied levels of support, addressing individual needs, in changing their physical activity patterns. Results from a feasibility study (N = 20) before the JR-SB study revealed that in general the intervention was well accepted by the participants because of its individual approach, that is, focusing on sedentary behavior–related goal-setting and behavioral choices in the individual participants' everyday life.[33] This individual focus is in accordance with the EULAR physical activity recommendations for IA, in which it is highlighted that where individual adaptations to general physical activity recommendations are needed, these should be based on a comprehensive assessment of physical, social, and psychological factors, including fatigue, pain, depression, and disease activity.[11]

Clinical Perspectives in Targeting Sedentary Behavior in Rheumatoid Arthritis

Generally, there is a broad understanding in clinical practice that physical activity is an important aspect of disease management in patients with RA.[11,15] However, research indicates that patients with IA perceive that health professionals often lack knowledge of the impact of physical activity and exercise on joint damage, thus sending "mixed messages" on physical activity and its benefits.[12] With new evidence emerging on sedentary behavior and the inverse relationship with health outcomes in RA,[27] the potential of increasing health professionals' knowledge of the full physical activity continuum in health promotion in RA is important. Hence, they would need to take on a broader clinical responsibility in disseminating and advocating reduction of sedentary behavior and replacing it with light-intensity physical activity supplementary to promoting daily MVPA. Potentially, health professionals and patients may find that increasing daily light physical activity overcomes the potential barriers for exercise and high-intensity physical activity in RA. Hence, reducing sitting time and replacing it with increased standing and stepping time is presumably manageable even on days when the patient is limited by RA-related symptoms, decreased physical function, and mobility.

SUMMARY

Although the health benefits associated with participating in MVPA are well recognized in patients with RA, this health behavior may not be a realistic goal for most patients. For this reason, a goal that focuses on reducing daily sitting time and increasing time spent in light-intensity physical activity may be suitable and still provide health benefits in patients with RA, although as of yet based on limited evidence. Methods to facilitate reduction of sedentary behavior in RA have not been fully explored. Studies that have reported some change in physical activity or sedentary behavior in patients with RA have often had an individual and behavioral approach, for instance, motivational interviewing, coaching, goal setting, feedback on behavior, and frequent contact with a health professional. Studies that investigate the full potential of using technology-based methods to change physical activity patterns in RA are needed, although it seems that text messages for encouraging physical activity levels in RA are promising. Aerobic exercise is still the most commonly advocated type of physical activity in RA, but the emerging evidence on replacing sedentary behavior with light physical activity will allow health professionals to target the full range of the physical activity continuum. Health professionals may benefit from education about behavior change techniques in promoting physical activity in RA.

REFERENCES

1. Baillet A, Zeboulon N, Gossec L, et al. Efficacy of cardiorespiratory aerobic exercise in rheumatoid arthritis: meta-analysis of randomized controlled trials. Arthritis Care Res (Hoboken) 2010;62(7):984–92.
2. Rongen-van Dartel SA, Repping-Wuts H, Flendrie M, et al. Effect of aerobic exercise training on fatigue in rheumatoid arthritis: a meta-analysis. Arthritis Care Res (Hoboken) 2015;67(8):1054–62.
3. Stavropoulos-Kalinoglou A, Metsios GS, Veldhuijzen van Zanten JJ, et al. Individualised aerobic and resistance exercise training improves cardiorespiratory fitness and reduces cardiovascular risk in patients with rheumatoid arthritis. Ann Rheum Dis 2013;72(11):1819–25.
4. Manns PJ, Dunstan DW, Owen N, et al. Addressing the nonexercise part of the activity continuum: a more realistic and achievable approach to activity programming for adults with mobility disability? Phys Ther 2012;92(4):614–25.
5. Pinto AJ, Roschel H, de Sa Pinto AL, et al. Physical inactivity and sedentary behavior: overlooked risk factors in autoimmune rheumatic diseases? Autoimmun Rev 2017;16(7):667–74.
6. Caspersen CJ, Powell KE, Christenson GM. Physical activity, exercise, and physical fitness: definitions and distinctions for health-related research. Public Health Rep 1985;100(2):126–31.
7. Sedentary Behaviour Research Network. Letter to the editor: standardized use of the terms "sedentary" and "sedentary behaviours". Appl Physiol Nutr Metab 2012;37(3):540–2.
8. Ainsworth BE, Haskell WL, Whitt MC, et al. Compendium of physical activities: an update of activity codes and MET intensities. Med Sci Sports Exerc 2000;32(9 Suppl):S498–504.
9. World Health Organization. Global recommendations on physical activity for health. Geneva (Switzerland): World Health Organization; 2010.
10. Iversen MD, Brawerman M, Iversen CN. Recommendations and the state of the evidence for physical activity interventions for adults with rheumatoid arthritis: 2007 to present. Int J Clin Rheumtol 2012;7(5):489–503.

11. Rausch Osthoff AK, Niedermann K, Braun J, et al. 2018 EULAR recommendations for physical activity in people with inflammatory arthritis and osteoarthritis. Ann Rheum Dis 2018;77(9):1251–60.
12. Verhoeven F, Tordi N, Prati C, et al. Physical activity in patients with rheumatoid arthritis. Joint Bone Spine 2016;83(3):265–70.
13. Larkin L, Gallagher S, Cramp F, et al. Behaviour change interventions to promote physical activity in rheumatoid arthritis: a systematic review. Rheumatol Int 2015; 35(10):1631–40.
14. Wilcox S, Der AC, Abbott J, et al. Perceived exercise barriers, enablers, and benefits among exercising and nonexercising adults with arthritis: results from a qualitative study. Arthritis Rheum 2006;55(4):616–27.
15. McKenna S, Kelly G, Kennedy N. A survey of physiotherapists' current management and the promotion of physical activity, in people with rheumatoid arthritis. Disabil Rehabil 2018;1–9 [Epub ahead of print].
16. Sokka T, Hakkinen A, Kautiainen H, et al. Physical inactivity in patients with rheumatoid arthritis: data from twenty-one countries in a cross-sectional, international study. Arthritis Rheum 2008;59(1):42–50.
17. Prioreschi A, Hodkinson B, Avidon I, et al. The clinical utility of accelerometry in patients with rheumatoid arthritis. Rheumatology (Oxford) 2013;52(9):1721–7.
18. Legge A, Blanchard C, Hanly JG. Physical activity and sedentary behavior in patients with systemic lupus erythematosus and rheumatoid arthritis. Open Access Rheumatol 2017;9:191–200.
19. Huffman KM, Pieper CF, Hall KS, et al. Self-efficacy for exercise, more than disease-related factors, is associated with objectively assessed exercise time and sedentary behaviour in rheumatoid arthritis. Scand J Rheumatol 2015; 44(2):106–10.
20. Hallal PC, Andersen LB, Bull FC, et al. Global physical activity levels: surveillance progress, pitfalls, and prospects. Lancet 2012;380(9838):247–57.
21. Thomsen T, Beyer N, Aadahl M, et al. Sedentary behaviour in patients with rheumatoid arthritis: a qualitative study. Int J Qual Stud Health Well-being 2015;10: 28578.
22. Biswas A, Oh PI, Faulkner GE, et al. Sedentary time and its association with risk for disease incidence, mortality, and hospitalization in adults: a systematic review and meta-analysis. Ann Intern Med 2015;162(2):123–32.
23. Wilmot EG, Edwardson CL, Achana FA, et al. Sedentary time in adults and the association with diabetes, cardiovascular disease and death: systematic review and meta-analysis. Diabetologia 2012;55(11):2895–905.
24. Grontved A, Hu FB. Television viewing and risk of type 2 diabetes, cardiovascular disease, and all-cause mortality: a meta-analysis. JAMA 2011;305(23):2448–55.
25. Healy GN, Dunstan DW, Salmon J, et al. Television time and continuous metabolic risk in physically active adults. Med Sci Sports Exerc 2008;40(4):639–45.
26. Ekelund U, Steene-Johannessen J, Brown WJ, et al. Does physical activity attenuate, or even eliminate, the detrimental association of sitting time with mortality? A harmonised meta-analysis of data from more than 1 million men and women. Lancet 2016;388(10051):1302–10.
27. Fenton SAM, Veldhuijzen van Zanten JJCS, Kitas GD, et al. Sedentary behaviour is associated with increased long-term cardiovascular risk in patients with rheumatoid arthritis independently of moderate-to-vigorous physical activity. BMC Musculoskelet Disord 2017;18(1):131.

28. Healy GN, Wijndaele K, Dunstan DW, et al. Objectively measured sedentary time, physical activity, and metabolic risk: the Australian Diabetes, Obesity and Lifestyle Study (AusDiab). Diabetes Care 2008;31(2):369–71.
29. Aadahl M, Linneberg A, Moller TC, et al. Motivational counseling to reduce sitting time: a community-based randomized controlled trial in adults. Am J Prev Med 2014;47(5):576–86.
30. Otten JJ, Jones KE, Littenberg B, et al. Effects of television viewing reduction on energy intake and expenditure in overweight and obese adults: a randomized controlled trial. Arch Intern Med 2009;169(22):2109–15.
31. Neuhaus M, Healy GN, Dunstan DW, et al. Workplace sitting and height-adjustable workstations: a randomized controlled trial. Am J Prev Med 2014; 46(1):30–40.
32. Alkhajah TA, Reeves MM, Eakin EG, et al. Sit-stand workstations: a pilot intervention to reduce office sitting time. Am J Prev Med 2012;43(3):298–303.
33. Thomsen T, Aadahl M, Beyer N, et al. Motivational counselling and SMS-reminders for reduction of daily sitting time in patients with rheumatoid arthritis: a descriptive randomised controlled feasibility study. BMC Musculoskelet Disord 2016;17(1):434.
34. Thomsen T, Aadahl M, Beyer N, et al. The efficacy of motivational counselling and SMS reminders on daily sitting time in patients with rheumatoid arthritis: a randomised controlled trial. Ann Rheum Dis 2017;76(9):1603–6.
35. Hetland ML. DANBIO–powerful research database and electronic patient record. Rheumatology (Oxford) 2011;50(1):69–77.
36. Epstein LH, Roemmich JN. Reducing sedentary behavior: role in modifying physical activity. Exerc Sport Sci Rev 2001;29(3):103–8.
37. Bandura A. Health promotion by social cognitive means. Health Educ Behav 2004;31(2):143–64.
38. Miller NH. Motivational interviewing as a prelude to coaching in healthcare settings. J Cardiovasc Nurs 2010;25(3):247–51.
39. Thomsen A, et al. The efficacy of motivational counselling and SMS-reminders on daily sitting time in patients with rheumatoid arthritis: 22 months follow-up of a randomised, parallel-group trial. Abstract to European League against Rheumatism (EULAR) congress, 2018.
40. Gilbert AL, Lee J, Ehrlich-Jones L, et al. A randomized trial of a motivational interviewing intervention to increase lifestyle physical activity and improve self-reported function in adults with arthritis. Semin Arthritis Rheum 2018;47(5): 732–40.
41. Martin A, Fitzsimons C, Jepson R, et al. Interventions with potential to reduce sedentary time in adults: systematic review and meta-analysis. Br J Sports Med 2015;49(16):1056–63.
42. Khoja SS, Almeida GJ, Wasko MC, et al. Light intensity physical activity is associated with lower cardiovascular risk factor burden in rheumatoid arthritis. Arthritis Care Res (Hoboken) 2015;68(4):424–31.
43. Knittle K, De Gucht V, Hurkmans E, et al. Targeting motivation and self-regulation to increase physical activity among patients with rheumatoid arthritis: a randomised controlled trial. Clin Rheumatol 2015;34(2):231–8.
44. Knittle K, De Gucht V, Hurkmans E, et al. Explaining physical activity maintenance after a theory-based intervention among patients with rheumatoid arthritis: process evaluation of a randomized controlled trial. Arthritis Care Res (Hoboken) 2016;68(2):203–10.

45. Griffiths AJ, White CM, Thain PK, et al. The effect of interactive digital interventions on physical activity in people with inflammatory arthritis: a systematic review. Rheumatol Int 2018;38(9):1623–34.
46. Hall AK, Cole-Lewis H, Bernhardt JM. Mobile text messaging for health: a systematic review of reviews. Annu Rev Public Health 2015;36:393–415.
47. Judice PB, Hamilton MT, Sardinha LB, et al. Randomized controlled pilot of an intervention to reduce and break-up overweight/obese adults' overall sitting-time. Trials 2015;16(1):490.
48. Nordgren B, Friden C, Demmelmaier I, et al. An outsourced health-enhancing physical activity program for people with rheumatoid arthritis: study of the maintenance phase. J Rheumatol 2018;45(8):1093–100.
49. Owen N, Salmon J, Koohsari MJ, et al. Sedentary behaviour and health: mapping environmental and social contexts to underpin chronic disease prevention. Br J Sports Med 2014;48(3):174–7.
50. Bakrania K, Edwardson CL, Bodicoat DH, et al. Associations of mutually exclusive categories of physical activity and sedentary time with markers of cardiometabolic health in English adults: a cross-sectional analysis of the Health Survey for England. BMC Public Health 2016;16:25.

Digital Patient Education and Decision Aids

Maria A. Lopez-Olivo, MD, PhD, Maria E. Suarez-Almazor, MD, PhD*

KEYWORDS

• Patient education • Decision aids • Digital tools • Multimedia tools
• Rheumatic diseases

KEY POINTS

- Patient education tools and decision aids can be developed and stored as digital data and delivered electronically with video or audio players, computers, or mobile devices.
- Digital patient education and decision aids can be tailored to facilitate health decision making and may benefit patient health outcomes.
- Digital patient education and decision aids should be based on evidence and must undergo a rigorous development and testing process.

INTRODUCTION

Consumer-informed health decision making includes several elements: understanding of the disease of interest; knowledge of related health care alternatives, including benefits, risks, and uncertainties; consideration of individual preferences; participation in decision making according to the role wanted to play (ie, passive, active, or collaborative); and making a decision consistent with individual values.[1,2] Shared decision making is a subset of informed decision making, with health care providers and patients working in partnership to determine the course of care most aligned with patients' values, which is the hallmark of patient-centered care. The Informed Medical Decisions Foundation defines shared decision making as a "collaborative process that allows patients (and families) and their providers (and the health care team) to make health care decisions together, taking into account the best scientific evidence available, as well as the patient's values and preferences. It honors both the provider's expert knowledge and the patient's right to be fully informed of all care options and the potential harms and benefits."[3] The shared decision-making process offers patients

Disclosure Statement: None.
Funding/Support: None.
Section of Rheumatology and Clinical Immunology, Division of Internal Medicine, Department of General Internal Medicine, The University of Texas MD Anderson Cancer Center, Unit 1465, 1515 Holcombe Boulevard, Houston, TX 77030, USA
* Corresponding author.
E-mail address: msalmazor@mdanderson.org

Rheum Dis Clin N Am 45 (2019) 245–256
https://doi.org/10.1016/j.rdc.2019.01.001
rheumatic.theclinics.com

the help they need to make the best individualized care choices, while enabling rheumatologists to feel certain about their recommendations.[4] A collaborative participation of patients in the decision-making process has been shown to increase trust, enhance realistic perceptions of risk and treatment expectations, improve clinical and patient-reported outcomes, and increase satisfaction and treatment adherence.[5,6] The first step in this complex process is acquiring the knowledge that can support preference-based and value-based decisions, which can be achieved through carefully developed evidence-based educational tools.

EVIDENCE-BASED PATIENT EDUCATION

There is a clear distinction between providing health information alone versus health education. Whereas information refers to the delivery of health-related facts to patients, health education is more complex and encompasses a systematic instruction that promotes an understanding on how to maintain personal health. Although patient education materials can be extremely useful, they also can be counterproductive if they include erroneous information, confuse the patient, or contradict consensus recommendations. For instance, imbalanced, poor-quality information about therapy where only an overoptimistic view is presented may result in requests for interventions that may not be suitable or in unexpected harms.[7]

Evidence-based patient education is the joint use of current medical best evidence to inform patients about their health and management options.[8] In 2008, the guidelines of the General Medical Council defined principles for the content of evidence-based patient education.[9] Patients should be informed about their diagnosis and prognosis, diagnostic uncertainties, management options, purpose of treatment and its potential benefits, risks, and associated burdens; understand who the people are involved in their care and their roles; and know their right to refuse treatment or seek a second opinion. Patient health education also should be transparent. Details about the purpose and sources of information and conflicts of interest should be provided.[8] Additionally, evidence-based patient education should be tailored according to patients' needs, wishes, and priorities; the nature of their condition; and the complexity of the treatment and associated risks. Individuals make decisions with respect to health issues according to how the problem and alternatives for solutions are presented to them.[10]

A growing array of approaches is available to address patients' educational needs and to encourage them to actively participate in managing their health issues. Patient education can improve knowledge; promote understanding of the disease (eg, prognosis, risk factors, and harms and benefits of interventions); improve cognitive skills, such as problem-solving and self-efficacy; and facilitate communication.[11] Individual knowledge, beliefs, and affects are brought to medical encounters and can influence patient-provider interactions. In addition, external influences from family and social networks also can play a role in health decisions. Health education should aim to model patients' expectancies of benefits and barriers, considering the various external influences from health care providers and social environment, to enhance beneficial behaviors, such as self-care and adherence, which can ultimately improve outcomes.[12]

DECISION AIDS

Decision aids are tools to inform patients who want to actively participate in health decision making and help them with explicit choices. These tools are most effective when used together with the counseling of a health care provider. They provide information about a health condition using the latest quality-rated scientific evidence and the options and outcomes regarding diagnosis and treatment of the condition and help clarify patients' personal values and understanding of the relative importance of the benefits and risks of options.[13,14]

Decision aids are important for patients with rheumatologic conditions, who are frequently asked to make complex decisions about their treatment. Often, the optimal course may be uncertain, and individual preferences are central to decision making, because factors, such as risk tolerance and symptom burden, may vary from person to person. A recent review concluded that, compared with usual care, people who use decision aids feel more knowledgeable and better informed about their values and have more active roles in decision making.[15] The review also demonstrated knowledge improvement and correct risk perceptions when decision aids are used in preparation or within consultations. Evidence suggests that these tools can be useful for a variety of clinical purposes and topics.

To deliver health education or decision aids effectively to patients affected by chronic conditions, it is important to understand their preferences with regard to their health information–seeking behavior. A study exploring the preferences of people living with different rheumatologic conditions for delivery methods of educational material found that for patients, the preferred media for obtaining treatment information were electronic media (televisions and DVDs) in their homes, doctors' offices, or pharmacy.[16] The preferred messengers were patients with the same disease and rheumatologists using real-life stories and testimonials, narrating both successful outcomes and failures. Key message topics preferred by patients included healthy lifestyle changes and benefits and consequences of medication adherence.[16]

DIGITAL PATIENT EDUCATION AND DECISION AIDS

The word, *digital*, describes items using binary digits (digital codes). When applied to patient education and decision aids, it usually relates to media stored as digital data, that is, software and platforms for teaching and learning that can be used with video or audio players, computers, or mobile devices. Different types of digital consumer and patient health tools are increasingly being developed to be delivered through electronic devices, such as computers and smartphones, as standalone software or Web sites.

With the rapid development of the Internet, digital technology has become a conventional method of health education for patients. It provides tremendous flexibility for delivering health information because Web sites and a broad range of applications can combine text, images, digital media such as audio and video, social networking tools, online games, animation, risk calculators and other interactive and personalized features that can help patients to think about their preferences and the role they want to play during the medical encounter. These tools can be delivered at a time and place that is chosen by an individual or a group of people simultaneously.

Advantages and Disadvantages

Digital patient education and decision aids bring new opportunities and challenges.[17] If the summary of decisions taken or education delivered is integrated with the patient electronic health record, data can be recorded longitudinally and reassessed and enhanced to make changes as needed, which could improve efficiency in patient-provider communications and better serve patient education needs. Because digital tools can include interactive features added to traditional media, such as text, graphics, or static images, and can be tailored individually, the information provided may better satisfy the needs and literacy levels of different populations. Because digital tools offer the convenience of accessibility, individuals have the choice to consult information almost anywhere, at any given time, and in relation to a topic of interest at that time.[17] Digital tools also can be visually appealing and entertaining and can include storylines and interactive elements, and patients may be more likely to engage cognitively and peruse and interpret the materials in their entirety compared with pencil-and-paper tools.[18]

Provision of digital tools alone does not necessarily ensure improved communication between clinicians and patients about treatment alternatives. There are practical barriers to using these tools, such as (1) providers resisting their use in practice because of the time required, causing disruption to clinic workflows; (2) with tools that are extensive, patients not taking the time to read or view them; and (3) tools that are costly to develop and difficult to disseminate having limits to their accessibility.[19] In addition, digital tools may require a degree of technical and health literacy. Poor health literacy has a disproportionate impact on patients with low education levels, those who belong to minority groups, and those who are elderly.[20] Individuals with limited health literacy often lack knowledge about their disease or misunderstand alternatives for treatment. Without this knowledge, they cannot participate in informed decision making about their health care options.[21–24] Studies in patients with rheumatic diseases have shown that those who had not completed high school had worse disease states than patients who had completed high school and that a low education level was a risk factor of premature death over a 10-year period.[25,26] Digital tools are commonly developed in English, containing data and navigation features that may be difficult for individuals with inadequate literacy or non-English speakers. There are scarce data on using digital patient education and decision aids in underserved populations.[27]

Development standards

Digital patient education and decision aid development are multifaceted, generally requiring prior theoretic and empirical groundwork.[28] Because the use of digital patient education and decision aids may have an impact in patient outcomes, a rigorous development process is required. Various instruments and checklists are available to evaluate the quality of patient education and decision aids. These apply to both non-digital and digital tools, although technical elements may be more relevant for the latter.

Since the release of the General Medical Council guidelines, various checklists have been developed to improve the quality of health patient information in general, adding new features to be evaluated, including accessibility, readability, comprehensiveness, design and layout, currency, strength of evidence, and relevance, among others. Based on a systematic review, the quality evaluation criteria for patient health information on the Internet should address 7 domains that are believed a minimum requirement: (1) accuracy (ie, information should be based on current guidelines or standards of care), (2) completeness/comprehensiveness (ie, covering the main concepts of the topic and subdivided to improve understanding), (3) technical elements (eg, sources of information, sponsorship, target audience, and so forth), (4) readability, (5) design and aesthetics (ie, elements to catch attention of visitors, such as layout, font type and size, and so forth), (6) accessibility (ie, content that can be used by a wide range of people living with disabilities), and (7) usability (ie, features to ease navigation).[29] Siddhanamatha and colleagues[30] conducted a study in 2017 evaluating a sample of health educational Web sites for rheumatoid arthritis and found that no Web site covered all needed information (ie, epidemiology, pathogenesis, treatment and disease monitoring, complications, self-management, risks and benefits of treatment, prognosis, treatment adherence, questions for patients to ask their doctors, and costs). The authors also identified problems with the reporting of important development information, such as when the content was last updated and the navigation experience. Most importantly, the mean reading level of the Web sites was above grade 12, which may render much of the information provided difficult to understand for patients with low literacy.[30]

Currently, there are no standards for digital decision aids; however, various quality evaluation criteria exist for decision aids in general, such as the International Patient Decision Aid Standards Collaboration assessment checklist; Workbook on Developing and Evaluating Patient Decision Aids, which evaluates the development and evaluation processes of decision aids; and Ensuring Quality Information for Patients, which evaluates information quality.[31–34] These instruments and checklists assess if the decision aid (1) provides information in sufficient detail, (2) presents probabilities in an unbiased manner, (3) includes methods to clarify values and preferences, (4) provides structured guidance for deliberation and communication, (5) presents information in balanced manner, (6) uses a systematic development process, (7) uses up-to-date evidence, (8) discloses conflicts of interest, (9) uses plain language, and (10) ensures that the decision is informed and values-based. Furthermore, in 2016, The National Quality Forum also published national standards for the certification of patient decision aids.[35] The set of performance measures assess the quality of shared decision making (**Box 1**).

Recently, a systematic review identified 6 features with different subcomponents that can be integrated in computer-based decision aids: (1) content control, described as the control a patient has over access to information, including navigation, clarity of information, optional information, and access to external sources; (2) tailoring, defined as the perception of the personal information received, including demographics, clinical condition, values, preferences and belief, and knowledge deficits; (3) patient narratives, a feature that allows patients to reflect on experiences of others either by using patient stories (with focus on personal experience) or behavior modeling (with focus on process deliberation); (4) values clarification, which is a process that helps patients examine personal values and preferences using decision points, notebooks, weighting or trade-off exercises, social matching, or personal reflection; (5) feedback-entailed interaction with the decision aid, including decision aid progress, knowledge, summary of preferences, optimal choice (using an algorithm/calculator), decisional consistency, and printed summary of decision aid activity; and (6) social support, described as encouraging patients to involve others in decision making, such as community support, integration of family, or facilitation of shared decision making; using questions for physicians, summary of decision aid in electronic health record, or video coaching to overcome physician communication barriers. The features found to improve the quality of decision making were content control, which allows patients to select the order, level of detail, and type of information presented; values clarification exercises, such as using notebooks to annotate the unclear topics or concerns, and trade-off exercises; overall feedback—an exception being the use of decisional consistency, which may give the impression that the initial decision was wrong and provoke negative emotions; and social support. In contrast, tailoring and patient narratives were associated with reduced quality of decision making.[36]

Given that the use of digital technologies for health education is rapidly evolving field, quality evaluation criteria will likely progress to incorporate elements more unique to digital tools, such as interaction, optimal navigation, and use in routine clinical practice.

Box 1
Certifying criteria intended to assist in determining the level to which a decision aid facilitates decision making

1. Provides a balanced presentation of options
2. Content is based on a rigorous and documented evidence synthesis method
3. Provides information about the evidence sources used
4. Provides key outcome probabilities, adopting risk communication principles
5. Provides a publication date
6. Provides information about the update policy and next expected update
7. Provides information about the funding sources used for development
8. Provides information about competing interests and/or policy
9. Provides information about the development process, including information about participation from target users and health professionals
10. Provides information about user testing with target patients and health professionals
11. Reports readability levels
12. Follows plain language guidelines, to ensure understanding of people with low literacy and/or low health literacy skills

Additional information required for screening and diagnostic tests

1. Describe what the test is designed to measure.
2. Describe next steps taken if a test detects a condition/problem.
3. Describe next steps if no condition/problem detected.
4. Describe consequences of detection that would not have caused problems if the screen were not done.
5. Include information on the test's positive predictive value.
6. Include information on the test's negative predictive value.

Data from Data National Quality Forum. National Standards for the Certification of Patient Decision Aids. Available at: https://www.qualityforum.org/Publications/2016/12/National_Standards_for_the_Certification_of_Patient_Decision_Aids.aspx.

Examples in rheumatology The studies described in this article do not represent an exhaustive review of this topic but rather are examples of controlled trials in different diseases comparing different delivery methods of patient education materials and decision aids. Although adding digital features may improve outcomes compared with reading materials alone, increasing levels of complexity are not always beneficial.

Increasingly, multimedia tools are being developed to provide health education to patients with rheumatic disorders. Many of these tools include audiovisual components, often with patient or clinician narratives, and they can incorporate storytelling (telenovela format). These interventions can be delivered in external devices, such as DVDs, or through the Internet. The authors have developed 3 multimedia video tools for patients with rheumatoid arthritis, osteoarthritis of the knee, and osteoporosis. The tools were designed to be didactic and entertaining, with simple navigation and graphic user interfaces, provided in both English and Spanish languages. The videos incorporate a series of soap opera segments depicting a main character with the disease of interest, integrated with learning modules to provide patients with factual information about their condition and treatment options, and also including patient testimonials. After viewing the tool, most participants believed they gained clarity on aspects related to disease course, symptoms, and the time medication takes to start acting; they were "encouraged to see their doctor regularly"; and they were more aware about taking their medications.[37]

A group randomized trial evaluated a 13-minute video that included patient stories related to their experiences with nonsteroidal anti-inflammatory drugs (NSAIDs), related adverse effects, and the importance of patient-provider communication.[38] The primary outcomes were the proportion of patients who spoke with their physician about NSAIDs used and their risks. The results showed that this intervention, primarily including patient stories, did not increase patient-physician interactions.

Several studies also have been conducted to evaluate multimedia and digital tools in patients requiring bone health care. This is an important area, because it has been extensively documented that rates for osteoporosis screening and treatment are universally low, despite well-publicized national guidelines.[39,40] Two parallel, group-randomized, controlled trials were conducted to evaluate the effectiveness of 2 interventions designed to increase appropriate dual-energy x-ray absorptiometry (DXA) and osteoporosis treatment in women greater than or equal to 65 years old.[41] Participants were allocated to 3 groups, each with a different strategy: (1) a system that permitted individuals to schedule their own DXA; (2) the self-schedule strategy combined with education that included a video containing narrative storytelling and written information to encourage patients to schedule a DXA and to encourage communication with their providers; and (3) a control group in which individuals needed to obtain authorization to schedule a DXA. The investigators concluded that DXA uptake was greater in the intervention groups compared with the usual care group; however, the addition of educational material to the self-schedule strategy did not provide a greater uptake.

A subsequent study by this group evaluated a multimodal intervention delivered via Internet and a DVD with relevant information for postmenopausal women with prior fracture.[42] The intervention incorporated print and audiovisual components (ie, patient narratives) and contained information individualized to the barriers or concerns expressed about osteoporosis management and readiness to behavior change. Interactive voice-response phone messages also were delivered to encourage viewing the DVD. The investigators evaluated the determinants associated with online intervention uptake. Patients providing an e-mail address were most likely to access the intervention within 60 days. In contrast, a negative correlation was found with follow-up phone calls; patients were less likely to interact with the intervention if they received the phone reminders.

A study in patients with rheumatoid arthritis evaluated a Web-based decision support tool to inform patients with active disease about the risks and benefits of biologic therapy. Options were presented with probabilistic estimations of outcomes. The tool allowed patients to weigh attributes for explicit value clarification, and feedback was provided, including the tool's suggested optimal choice according to stated preferences.[43] The results showed an increase in knowledge, willingness to take a biologic, and informed value-concordant choices after completion of the tool. Recently, a Web-based educational intervention with interactive components was developed to educate first-degree relatives of patients with rheumatoid arthritis about their risk factors for developing this disease. The tool included a personalized risk estimator on the basis of demographics, genetics, autoantibodies, and behaviors.[44] The tool was successfully implemented and evaluated in a randomized controlled trial. Participants receiving the tool had increased, long-lasting knowledge on risk factors than controls after completion of the program.

Some studies in patients with rheumatic diseases have used more complex methodologies to develop decision aids. Conjoint analysis is a marketing methodology that is used to understand and aid in decision-making processes by determining how people value different attributes at different levels, by measuring the stated preferences of individuals.[45] These interactive tools help people select and rank how they value different attributes for a given product (in market research) or a health condition or intervention (in health research). By engaging in this preference exercise, individuals can compare and choose among multiattribute alternatives, in turn leading to an explicit values clarification, which can aid in decision making. A 2007 randomized controlled trial compared an Adaptive Conjoint Analysis (ACA) tool (Sawtooth Software, Provo, Utah, USA) developed with a commercial software for the treatment of knee pain with an informational pamphlet.[46] The intervention was designed to increase patient awareness of choices for available treatment options, including explicit values clarification delivered via trade-off exercises and feedback through summary of preferences, optimal choice, and a summary of the decision aid activity. The primary outcome was decisional self-efficacy. Participants using the digital tool trusted more in their ability to get information about existing options, felt better prepared to participate in their visit, and were more confident in managing their arthritis compared with patients receiving the information pamphlet only. A subsequent study by the same group compared 2 surveys in patients with knee pain, which described attributes related to pain, energy, route of administration, stomach upset, bleeding ulcer, and cost.[47] In the first survey, participants were presented all attributes and chose the most important one. In the second survey, they rated the importance of the remaining attributes relative to the one they had chosen to be the most important one. Both surveys performed well. Explicit value clarification tools can be valuable tools, which are easier to present in digital formats and can be incorporated in digital decision aids to elicit patient preferences and facilitate medical decision making.

The authors conducted a randomized controlled trial using adaptive conjoint analysis with the same software, this time in patients with osteoarthritis of the knee, to aid them in decision making related to total knee replacement.[48] Patients were randomized to receive 1 of the following: (1) educational booklet; (2) educational booklet combined with video booklet; or (3) educational booklet + video booklet + conjoint analysis exercise. The primary outcome was decisional conflict. Although all groups had a reduction in decisional conflicts, the largest reduction was observed in the group watching the video booklet, indicating that adding a more complex digital values clarification exercise did not increase the potential benefit of the educational tools. A qualitative study in a subset of this study group identified the concerns that elderly patients had using the conjoint analysis tool: some were confused by the series of comparisons, others believed the software did not adequately reflect the preferences expressed during its use, and many felt overwhelmed by the number of choices they were given.[49]

Although less studied than other features/components of digital patient education and decision aids, social support can be an important source of health information and can aid in decision making. A pilot randomized controlled trial evaluating a peer mentoring program through video chat application [or software] for adolescents with juvenile idiopathic arthritis found that participants' mean engagement level with the program was 8.5 of a maximum of 10. Participants who completed the program improved in their perceived ability to manage the disease compared with controls.[50] The authors recently completed a randomized controlled trial that compared patients with rheumatoid arthritis assigned to participate in a closed Facebook community, with guidance from an experience patient moderator, with patients who did not participate in the community and only had access to an educational Web site.[51] Although no differences were observed in gains in knowledge or self-efficacy, patients participating in the Facebook community reported increased satisfaction in peer support compared with nonparticipants.

SUMMARY

For many rheumatic conditions, decisions can be difficult both emotionally and cognitively, often including more than one clinically appropriate option, resulting in choices driven by personal values and preferences. A first step in decision making is knowledge of the available options and clear understanding of the relevant benefits, harms, and contextual factors associated with each alternative.

Over the past decade, patient education tools have been gradually moving toward digital platforms with preference toward the online, computer-based environment. The content provided in digital tools must conform to the highest standards of scientific accuracy, must be tested for comprehensibility and relevance, and adhere to national standards. Selecting evidence-based digital patient education, however, is not sufficient. It is equally important to know how and when the digital tool is presented to a patient.

Decision aids help patients engage in decision-making processes by providing the best available evidence of potential harms and benefits for different alternatives, so they can make informed, values-based decisions with their health care providers. Successful implementation of digital shared decision-making tools is complex and depends on key factors, such as a patient's health literacy, available evidence on the health topic of interest, and clinic-related issues (eg, time and competing priorities in the consultation).[52]

Finally, patient involvement in the development process of educational and decision tools is essential to ensure relevant content and usability. These issues will influence the potential benefit and satisfaction with the tool.

REFERENCES

1. Sheridan SL, Harris RP, Woolf SH, Shared Decision-Making Workgroup of the U.S. Preventive Services Task Force. Shared decision making about screening and chemoprevention. a suggested approach from the U.S. Preventive Services Task Force. Am J Prev Med 2004;26(1):56–66.
2. Briss P, Rimer B, Reilley B, et al. Promoting informed decisions about cancer screening in communities and healthcare systems. Am J Prev Med 2004;26(1): 67–80.
3. Informed Medical Decisions Foundation. What is shared decision making?. 2009. Available at: http://www.informedmedicaldecisions.org/. Accessed July 6, 2009.
4. Montori VM, Kunneman M, Hargraves I, et al. Shared decision making and the internist. Eur J Intern Med 2017;37:1–6.
5. Hauser K, Koerfer A, Kuhr K, et al. Outcome-relevant effects of shared decision making. Dtsch Arztebl Int 2015;112(40):665–71.
6. Joosten EA, DeFuentes-Merillas L, de Weert GH, et al. Systematic review of the effects of shared decision-making on patient satisfaction, treatment adherence and health status. Psychother Psychosom 2008;77(4):219–26.
7. Coulter A. Evidence based patient information. is important, so there needs to be a national strategy to ensure it. BMJ 1998;317(7153):225–6.
8. Bunge M, Muhlhauser I, Steckelberg A. What constitutes evidence-based patient information? Overview of discussed criteria. Patient Educ Couns 2010;78(3): 316–28.

9. General Medical Council. Consent: patients and doctors making decisions together. 2008. Available at: https://www.gmc-uk.org/ethical-guidance/ethical-guidance-for-doctors/consent. Accessed August 31, 2018.
10. Thaler RH, Sunstein CR. Nudge: improving decisions about health, wealth, and happiness. New Haven (CT): Yale University Press; 2009.
11. Zimmerman EB, Woolf SH, Haley A. Understanding the relationship between education and health: a review of the evidence and an examination of community perspectives. Rockville (MD): Agency for Healthcare Research and Quality; 2015. Available at: https://www.ahrq.gov/professionals/education/curriculum-tools/population-health/zimmerman.html.
12. Suarez-Almazor ME, Richardson M, Kroll TL, et al. A qualitative analysis of decision-making for total knee replacement in patients with osteoarthritis. J Clin Rheumatol 2010;16(4):158–63.
13. Selby JV, Beal AC, Frank L. The Patient-Centered Outcomes Research Institute (PCORI) national priorities for research and initial research agenda. JAMA 2012;307(15):1583–4.
14. Methodology Committee of the Patient-Centered Outcomes Research Institute (PCORI). Methodological standards and patient-centeredness in comparative effectiveness research: the PCORI perspective. JAMA 2012;307(15):1636–40.
15. Stacey D, Legare F, Lewis K, et al. Decision aids for people facing health treatment or screening decisions. Cochrane Database Syst Rev 2017;(4):CD001431.
16. Lopez-Olivo MA, Volk R, Jibaja-Weiss M, et al. Preferred strategies for delivering treatment information to people with rheumatoid arthritis, osteoarthritis and osteoporosis. Arthritis Rheum 2013;65:S419.
17. Ren W, Huang C, Liu Y, et al. The application of digital technology in community health education. Digit Med 2015;1:3–6. Available at: http://www.digitmedicine.com/article.asp?issn=2226-8561;year=2015;volume=1;issue=1;spage=3;epage=6;aulast=Ren. Accessed February 14, 2019.
18. Lam M, Choi M, Lam HR, et al. Use of multimedia in patient and caregiver education for cancer pain management: a literature review. Ann Palliat Med 2017;6(1):66–72.
19. Elwyn G, Rix A, Holt T, et al. Why do clinicians not refer patients to online decision support tools? Interviews with front line clinics in the NHS. BMJ Open 2012;2(6).
20. Paasche-Orlow MK, Parker RM, Gazmararian JA, et al. The prevalence of limited health literacy. J Gen Intern Med 2005;20(2):175–84.
21. Baker DW, Parker RM, Williams MV, et al. Health literacy and the risk of hospital admission. J Gen Intern Med 1998;13(12):791–8.
22. Baker DW, Gazmararian JA, Williams MV, et al. Functional health literacy and the risk of hospital admission among Medicare managed care enrollees. Am J Public Health 2002;92(8):1278–83.
23. Al Sayah F, Majumdar SR, Johnson JA. Association of inadequate health literacy with health outcomes in patients with type 2 diabetes and depression: secondary analysis of a controlled trial. Can J Diabetes 2015;39(4):259–65.
24. Schillinger D, Grumbach K, Piette J, et al. Association of health literacy with diabetes outcomes. JAMA 2002;288(4):475–82.
25. Rudd RE, Rosenfeld L, Gall V. Health literacy and arthritis research and practice. Curr Opin Rheumatol 2007;19(2):97–100.
26. Pincus T, Keysor J, Sokka T, et al. Patient questionnaires and formal education level as prospective predictors of mortality over 10 years in 97% of 1416 patients with rheumatoid arthritis from 15 United States private practices. J Rheumatol 2004;31(2):229–34.

27. Marrin K, Wood F, Firth J, et al. Option Grids to facilitate shared decision making for patients with Osteoarthritis of the knee: protocol for a single site, efficacy trial. BMC Health Serv Res 2014;14:160.
28. Lenz M, Buhse S, Kasper J, et al. Decision aids for patients. Dtsch Arztebl Int 2012;109(22–23):401–8.
29. Eysenbach G, Powell J, Kuss O, et al. Empirical studies assessing the quality of health information for consumers on the world wide web: a systematic review. JAMA 2002;287(20):2691–700.
30. Siddhanamatha HR, Heung E, Lopez-Olivo MLA, et al. Quality assessment of websites providing educational content for patients with rheumatoid arthritis. Semin Arthritis Rheum 2017;46(6):715–23.
31. International Patient Decision Aid Standards (IPDAS)Collaboration. International patient decision aid standards. Available at: http://ipdas.ohri.ca/. Accessed February 14, 2019.
32. O'Connor A, Jacobsen MJ. Workbook on developing and evaluating patient decision aids, 2003. Available at https://decisionaid.ohri.ca/docs/develop/develop_da.pdf. Accessed on February 14, 2019.
33. Lenz M, Kasper J. MATRIX - development and feasibility of a guide for quality assessment of patient decision aids. Psychosoc Med 2007;4:Doc09.
34. Moult B, Franck LS, Brady H. Ensuring quality information for patients: development and preliminary validation of a new instrument to improve the quality of written health care information. Health Expect 2004;7(2):165–75.
35. National Quality Forum. National Standards for the Certification of Patient Decision Aids. Available at: https://www.qualityforum.org/Publications/2016/12/National_Standards_for_the_Certification_of_Patient_Decision_Aids.aspx. Accessed February 14, 2019.
36. Syrowatka A, Kromker D, Meguerditchian AN, et al. Features of computer-based decision aids: systematic review, thematic synthesis, and meta-analyses. J Med Internet Res 2016;18(1):e20.
37. Lopez-Olivo MA, Ingleshwar A, Volk RJ, et al. Development and pilot testing of multimedia patient education tools for patients with knee osteoarthritis, osteoporosis, and rheumatoid arthritis. Arthritis Care Res (Hoboken) 2018;70(2):213–20.
38. Miller MJ, Weech-Maldonado R, Outman RC, et al. Evaluating the effectiveness of a patient storytelling DVD intervention to encourage physician-patient communication about nonsteroidal anti-inflammatory drug (NSAID) use. Patient Educ Couns 2016;99(11):1837–44.
39. McKenna JE, Melzack R. Analgesia produced by lidocaine microinjection into the dentate gyrus. Pain 1992;49(1):105–12.
40. Curtis JR, Carbone L, Cheng H, et al. Longitudinal trends in use of bone mass measurement among older americans, 1999-2005. J Bone Miner Res 2008; 23(7):1061–7.
41. Warriner AH, Outman RC, Feldstein AC, et al. Effect of self-referral on bone mineral density testing and osteoporosis treatment. Med Care 2014;52(8):743–50.
42. Danila MI, Outman RC, Rahn EJ, et al. A multi-modal intervention for Activating Patients at Risk for Osteoporosis (APROPOS): rationale, design, and uptake of online study intervention material. Contemp Clin Trials Commun 2016;4:14–24.
43. Fraenkel L, Peters E, Charpentier P, et al. Decision tool to improve the quality of care in rheumatoid arthritis. Arthritis Care Res (Hoboken) 2012;64(7):977–85.
44. Prado MG, Iversen MD, Yu Z, et al. Effectiveness of a web-based personalized rheumatoid arthritis risk tool with or without a health educator for knowledge of rheumatoid arthritis risk factors. Arthritis Care Res 2018;70(10):1421–30.

45. Ryan M, Farrar S. Using conjoint analysis to elicit preferences for health care. BMJ 2000;320(7248):1530–3.
46. Fraenkel L, Rabidou N, Wittink D, et al. Improving informed decision-making for patients with knee pain. J Rheumatol 2007;34(9):1894–8.
47. Fraenkel L. Feasibility of using modified adaptive conjoint analysis importance questions. Patient 2010;3(4):209–15.
48. de Achaval S, Fraenkel L, Volk RJ, et al. Impact of educational and patient decision aids on decisional conflict associated with total knee arthroplasty. Arthritis Care Res (Hoboken) 2012;64(2):229–37.
49. Rochon D, Eberth JM, Fraenkel L, et al. Elderly patients' experiences using adaptive conjoint analysis software as a decision aid for osteoarthritis of the knee. Health Expect 2014;17(6):840–51.
50. Stinson J, Ahola Kohut S, Forgeron P, et al. The iPeer2Peer Program: a pilot randomized controlled trial in adolescents with Juvenile Idiopathic Arthritis. Pediatr Rheumatol Online J 2016;14(1):48.
51. Lopez-Olivo MA, Foreman J, Lin H, et al. Effects of social networking on chronic disease management in rheumatoid arthritis [abstract]. Arthritis Rheumatol 2018;70(suppl 10). https://acrabstracts.org/abstract/effects-of-social-networking-on-chronic-disease-management-in-rheumatoid-arthritis/. Accessed February 14, 2019.
52. Nielson-Bohlman L, Panzer AM, Kindig DA. Health literacy: a prescription to end confusion. Washington, DC: The National Academies Press; 2004.

Using Health Information Technology to Support Use of Patient-Reported Outcomes in Rheumatology

Julie Gandrup, MD, Jinoos Yazdany, MD, MPH*

KEYWORDS

- Patient-reported outcomes • PROs • Health IT • eHealth • mHealth

KEY POINTS

- Well thought-out collection of electronic patient-reported outcomes (PROs) may bridge the gap between providers and patient perspectives by focusing the encounter more on the patient's experience and perceptions of disease impact.
- This review illustrates that a number of digital tools to collect PROs have been developed both within electronic health records and in freestanding applications, most focused on rheumatoid arthritis.
- Work to date demonstrates that attention to design, including workflow planning, consideration of user burden, integration into health–information technology ecosystems, and delivery of accurate and timely information are important to successful implementation.
- Tools must be tested in diverse health systems and populations to ensure they are simple to interpret, useful for clinical decision making, and effective in impacting outcomes.

INTRODUCTION

The growing measurement of patient-reported outcomes (PROs) combined with the increasing adoption of health information technology (IT) and electronic health records (EHRs) as a means of collecting PRO data at scale present an unprecedented opportunity for advancing the science and practice of rheumatology.[1] The standardization of electronic collection of PRO data and the incorporation of these data into routine

Disclosure Statement: This work was supported by R18 HS025638 from the Agency for Healthcare Research and Quality. Dr J. Yazdany is also supported by the Robert L. Kroc Endowed Chair in Rheumatic and Connective Tissue Diseases and the Russell/Engleman Rheumatology Research Center at the University of California, San Francisco. Dr J. Yazdany has received research funding support from Pfizer. The views expressed are those of the authors and do not reflect the official views of the Agency for Healthcare Research and Quality.
Division of Rheumatology, University of California, San Francisco, San Francisco, CA, USA
* Corresponding author. 1001 Potrero Avenue, Suite 3300, San Francisco, CA 94110.
E-mail address: Jinoos.yazdany@ucsf.edu

Rheum Dis Clin N Am 45 (2019) 257–273
https://doi.org/10.1016/j.rdc.2019.01.007
rheumatic.theclinics.com
0889-857X/19/

clinical practice is anticipated to move the field of rheumatology closer to its goal of providing high-quality, affordable care, in ways that matter most to patients.[2] In addition, by facilitating timely and effective use of PROs without unreasonably adding to clinic workload, health IT has potential to bridge the gap between health care providers and patient perspectives in rheumatology by focusing the clinical encounter more on individual patient perceptions of disease impact.

Although a great number of validated PROs are available and commonly deployed in clinical practice, particularly for rheumatoid arthritis (RA), clinical workflows to meaningfully incorporate these data to monitor disease trajectories, guide treatment decisions, engage patients in disease management, and improve the patient-centeredness of care are lagging.[3] Challenges remain in adequately and meaningfully leveraging these data in rheumatology, and few studies have examined the impact and feasibility of using health IT–based tools to standardize PRO collection during outpatient visits.[4,5]

In this article, we review experiences with existing electronic efforts to collect and evaluate electronic PRO data in routine practice. Our findings are drawn from a structured review of the literature and include examples from 2 different national electronic collection efforts, 1 in the United States and 1 in Denmark. We discuss the lessons learned from previous work using health IT tools integrated with the EHR or as stand-alone applications to collect PROs in clinical care in rheumatology. Finally, we frame an agenda for future work supporting ways to meaningfully leverage electronic collection of PROs to improve the patient-centeredness of rheumatologic care.

ELECTRONIC COLLECTION OF PATIENT-REPORTED OUTCOMES AT INDIVIDUAL CLINIC LEVEL

We performed a semistructured review of the literature (detailed in Appendix 1) to identify published health IT tools to collect PROs in clinical rheumatology settings in the past 10 years. We searched for both EHR-enabled tools and stand-alone applications to aid collection of PROs. Special attention was paid to the design process, adoption and integration into routine care, patient and physician satisfaction with use, and evaluation of patient outcomes after implementation. We excluded studies about pediatric or orthopedic management as well as self-monitoring tools without health care provider participation.

An overview of the 10 health IT tools identified and evaluated in our review can be found in **Table 1**. We review each of these electronic tools, categorized by mode of PRO collection and EHR integration status (**Fig. 1**), and discuss what challenges and opportunities each of these integration methods provide.

We found significant heterogeneity among the health IT–enabled PRO collection tools, which emphasizes the need for a general framework for systematic incorporation of the patient's perspective in routine clinical care. We also found that published reports of rigorous digital tools are relatively few, and they are predominantly designed for use in caring for patients with RA rather than other rheumatological conditions.

Stand-Alone Digital Tools

We identified several examples of stand-alone digital tools. These tools exist entirely outside of the EHR, and are accessed by patients as well as clinicians through online links or Web-based applications.

READY (RhEumAtic Disease activitY) is an app (iPad)-based stand-alone ePRO application that enables the PRO data capture process to occur at physician offices using a tablet.[6] It uses multiple validated PRO questionnaires that reflect symptoms

Table 1
Characteristics of electronic tools designed for PRO collection in clinical rheumatology

Reference	Tool/Intervention	Population (n)	EHR Integration	Mode of Collection	Outcome
Chua et al,[11] 2015	Electronic version of RAPID-3 questionnaire. Patients access it by logging into an online Patient Portal within 7 d of visit.	RA (68)	Yes	Patient portal	Validation of performance characteristics of EHR version of RAPID-3 compared with paper version
Collier et al,[10] 2009	Rheumatology OnCall (ROC). Facilitates access to data relevant to encounter, but located in separate parts of the EHR. Automatic calculation of DAS28 with a homunculus for joint counts.	RA (15 physicians)	Yes	Full EHR integration	Physician satisfaction based on weekly and close-out survey
Dixon et al,[14,15] 2016	REMORA. Remote electronic collection of PROs between clinic visits through an app. Data automatically integrates with the EHR.	RA (21)	Yes	Remote monitoring	Patient and physician satisfaction
Li et al,[13] 2018	Online Epic EHR patient portal accessible from home to collect PROMIS PF-10a within 7 d of visit.	RA (1078)	Yes	Patient portal	Comparison of proportion of visits with documented PROMIS PF scores across age, race and ethnicity, and language and examination of trends over time

(continued on next page)

Table 1
(*continued*)

Reference	Tool/Intervention	Population (n)	EHR Integration	Mode of Collection	Outcome
El Miedany et al,[7] 2010	Online PRO questionnaire accessible from any device the patient has available. Enables automatic collection of DAS28 and RAPID-3.	RA (211)	No	Web-based stand-alone	Equivalence of outcomes (RAPID-3 and DAS28) between electronic and paper formats; patients' medication adherence
Newman et al,[3] 2015	Rheum-PACER. Integrates information from 4 data sources and reassembles them into actionable views and functions during clinic visit. Facilitates automatic calculation of CDAI.	RA (6725)	Yes	Full EHR integration	Adoption (RAPID-3, CDAI), efficiency (time to review information), productivity (level of service and corresponding relative value units), and patient perception (patient activation, adherence, satisfaction)
Salaffi et al,[16] 2016	RETE-MARCHE. Telemonitoring system. Online platform to administer computerized questionnaires to collect RAID and CDAI.	RA (44)	No	Remote monitoring	Proportion of patients in clinical remission at 1 y (CDAI <2.8); radiographic progression; patient acceptance

Salaffi et al,[8] 2013	SPEAMonitor. Electronic touchscreen tablet to complete computerized versions of the BASFI and BASDAI.	Axial spondylo-arthritis (55)	No	Web-based stand-alone	Usability (in terms of patients' acceptance, preference, and reliability) of computer-based questionnaires; feasibility (time taken to complete electronic vs paper questionnaires)
Schougaard et al,[17] 2016	AmbuFlex. Clinical telePRO tool that provides clinical decision support to suggest whether an outpatient visit is necessary.	RA (not known)	Yes	Remote monitoring	Describe experiences with respect to PRO data collection, the PRO-based automated decision algorithm, and PRO-based graphical overview for clinical decision support
Yen et al,[6] 2016	READY. Tablet application to collect PROs in the waiting room. Uses multiple validated PRO questionnaires that reflect RA symptoms and quality of life.	Not disease-specific; tested in RA (33)	Partial[a]	Stand-alone	Usability evaluation (think-aloud) and a time-motion study to observe changes in clinical workflow

Abbreviations: BASDAI, Bath Ankylosing Spondylitis Disease Activity Index; BASFI, Bath Ankylosing Spondylitis Functional Index; CDAI, Clinical Disease Activity Index; EHR, electronic health record; PRO, patient-reported outcome; PROMIS PF, Patient-Reported Outcomes Measurement Information System, physical function; RA, rheumatoid arthritis; RAID, RA Impact of Disease; READY, RhEumAtic Disease activity; REMORA, REmote MOnitoring of Rheumatoid Arthritis.

[a] Integration with a commercial EHR vendor occurred after the manuscript was published.

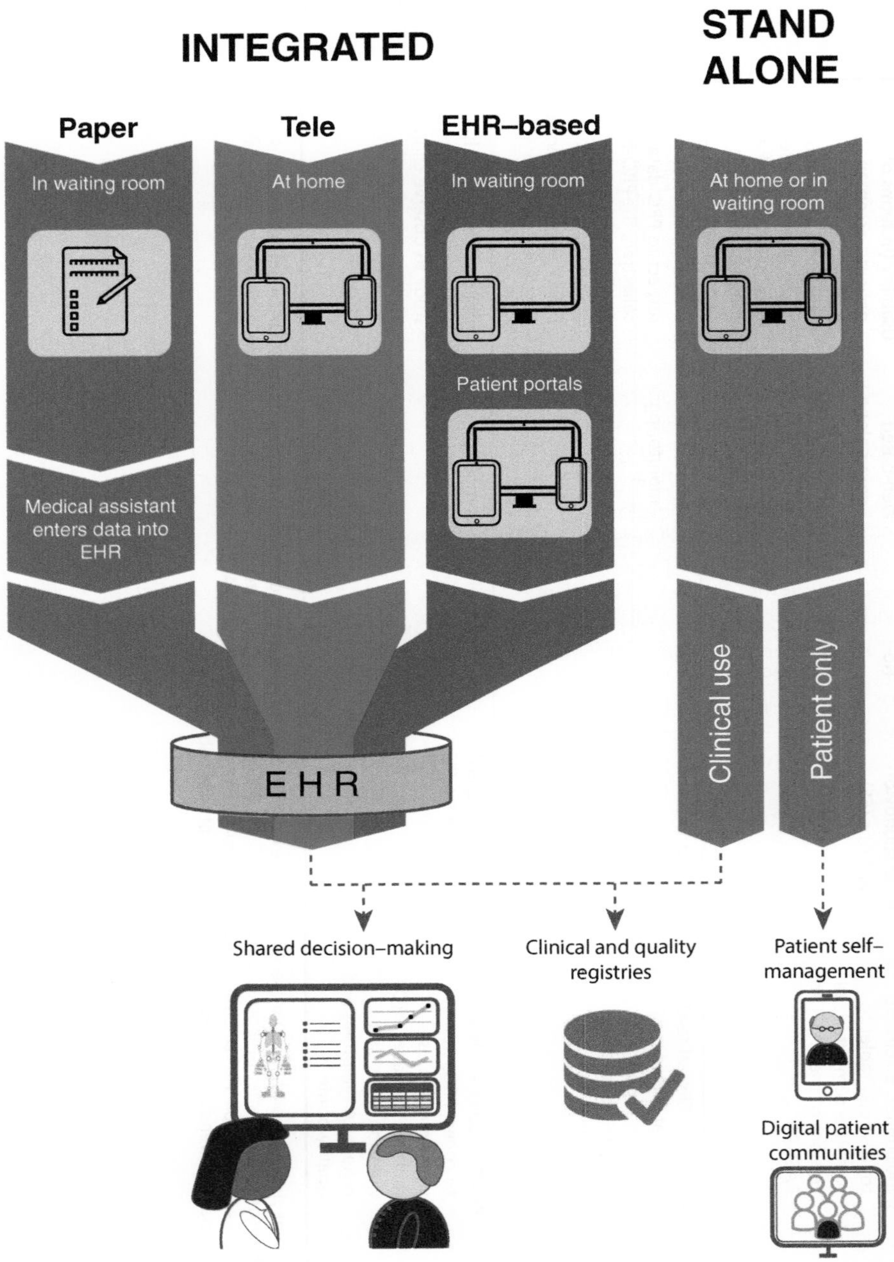

Fig. 1. Depiction of PRO landscape. From left to right: "Paper" collection entails the patient filling out PRO questionnaires in the waiting room, before medical assistant enters results into the EHR system. In "Tele" systems patients can deliver PROs via personal devices at their convenience, and data are automatically transferred to the EHR. "EHR-based" is similar to the tele solution, but patients either enter PROs in the waiting room before their encounter on devices linked directly to the clinic's EHR system or deliver PROs before their visits through the online patient portal. Finally, "stand-alone" tools are separate from the EHR system, and both patient and provider access questionnaires and results through an external online platform. Stand-alone systems additionally provide the opportunity for patients to monitor their PROs on personalized dashboards on their smartphone or feed data into online patient communities.

and quality of life of rheumatic diseases, with the option to show trended scores. Usability issues were found in READY, including touchscreen sensitivity (not sensitive enough when users attempted to complete an action), interface design (layout and font size), and instruction and error messages. Despite these issues, most patients with RA who tested the app found READY easier to use than the current PRO paper questionnaire. This was due mostly to the larger font size and the ease of "tapping" rather than writing-out or circling answers. Workflow and activity changes were observed in a time-motion study, and overall the tool did not extend the total time of patient visit.

El Miedany and colleagues[7] also developed a Web-based stand-alone system in which clinic staff manually entered ePROs into the EHR. A double-blinded, randomized controlled study including 211 patients with early RA was carried out. Patients were randomized to group 1, and completed an ePRO questionnaire monthly, or group 2, and continued to complete standard paper PROs. The primary endpoint was the difference in outcomes of RAPID-3 and DAS28 in both groups and secondary outcomes included medication adherence. After 12 months, there was no statistically significant difference in disease activity measures between the 2 groups. Based on pharmacy data, 89.6% of group 1 patients were adherent to their medications in comparison to 70.5% in the control group (*P*<.01). In group 1, fewer patients (5.7%) stopped medication because of intolerance compared with controls (19%). Unfortunately, it was unclear from the methods exactly how the collected PROs were implemented in clinical care or how they were acted on to reach these notable results.

In axial spondyloarthritis, a touchscreen tablet application for ePRO collection (SPEAMonitor) resulted in a lower mean amount of time spent completing the questionnaires (Bath Ankylosing Spondylitis Functional Index and Bath Ankylosing Spondylitis Disease Activity Index) than on paper (5.1 vs 7.9 minutes).[8,9] The tablet was also reported to be easier to use by patients, and age, computer experience, or education level did not influence results. The tool was designed to be user-friendly to patients by combining cartoon, writing, and voice and presenting only one question at a time. It was validated against a standard paper questionnaire and there was excellent score agreement. As only the validity of the tool was assessed, implementation into actual clinical workflow was not discussed.

Fully Integrated Electronic Health Record–Based Tool

Several studies examined tools that were fully integrated with an EHR. Full integration involves developing methods to capture key PRO data elements in structured fields within the EHR (just as vital signs or laboratory tests are currently captured).

The Rheum-PACER software integrates and reassembles information from the patient (via a touchscreen questionnaire), nurse, physician, and Epic EHR into a series of actionable views in an application outside the EHR, while feeding information back to the EHR. Core functions include tools to facilitate documentation of key aspects of RA care for patient and provider and graphical displays to examine outcome trends over time. The tool was integrated and tested in 3 rheumatology clinics. Over 2 years, 86% of patients and rheumatologists used the software. Physician-reported chart review time decreased from a median of 5 minutes before Rheum-PACER to 4 minutes after Rheum-PACER and implementation and documentation time decreased from a median of 7 to 5.5 minutes, although neither reached statistical significance. In addition, a strong, significant correlation was seen between physician use of the software and disease control (weighted Pearson correlation coefficient 0.59), and the investigators showed a relative increase in patients with low disease activity of 3% per quarter.[3]

Similarly, the Rheumatology OnCall (ROC) application gathered rheumatology-pertinent data from laboratory, microbiology, pathology, radiology, and pharmacy information systems within the EHR, and also included a disease activity calculator.[10] In total, 15 rheumatologists (of 47 in the clinic) accessed ROC during outpatient visits at the time of the clinical encounter. Trended clinical and laboratory data populated a dashboard that allowed the clinician to quickly assess trends and facilitated the tracking of disease activity. The investigators also conducted a 12-week prospective cohort study to assess physicians' attitudes toward use. By administering weekly physician surveys, they demonstrated that most physicians found graphing trends useful. In a close-out survey, the most physicians reported that use of ROC improved patient care, and that they would continue to use ROC in daily RA patient care. However, the frequency of use of the ROC was inconsistent among physicians, pointing to general barriers to health IT adoption. No objective assessment of patient outcomes was carried out. Planned enhancements to the application include disease activity calculators for systemic lupus erythematosus, ankylosing spondylitis, and osteoarthritis.

Patient Portals Within the Electronic Health Record

Similar to fully integrated tools, 2 studies examined the use of online EHR patient portals to collect ePROs. These portals permit patients to retrieve their health records and to enter additional information available to the clinician. Chua and colleagues[11,12] prompted patients with RA to complete an online version of the RAPID 3 via the patient portal anytime in the week before their upcoming appointment. The EHR automatically calculated and interpreted the disease activity score for the electronic RAPID 3, and prior scores could be easily accessed to facilitate comparisons. The study mainly focused on validating the electronic RAPID 3 compared with the paper version and they found no statistical difference by collection method. Limitations included the lack of a qualitative component to the study to help understand patients' personal experiences in terms of acceptance, convenience, and preference when answering the online questionnaires. In addition, only 52.5% of the clinic's 1130 patients with RA had an active EHR patient portal, possibly representing a subpopulation of patients more comfortable with using technology.

Li and colleagues[13] likewise assessed the collection of PROs from patients with RA using a paper version and an online form through an Epic EHR patient portal (MyChart). Patients with an activated portal received a message 7 days before their appointment with a link to the PROMIS (Patient-Reported Outcomes Measurement Information System) physical function (PF) form. They examined the proportion of patients completing the form electronically or on paper and explored patient factors associated with method of completion. One and a half years after the online patient portal survey became available, only 19.3% of visits had an associated online PROMIS PF score, and no patients used it persistently; more than half of patients abandoned the online portal for PRO reporting after a single use. In addition, the investigators showed that use lagged among racial and ethnic minorities. Online portal use did not decrease the burden of data collection and data entry for staff as anticipated, because the clinic workflow still required that medical assistants assessed whether a patient already completed an online version of the survey at the time of patient check-in. This process was time-consuming and faulty, as evidenced by the numerous patients who completed both online and paper surveys within 7 days of an in-person visit. Limitations included the lack of data collection regarding patients' home Internet and computer access as well as health literacy level, which might have explained low uptake in some groups. Issues of portal access, enrollment, satisfaction, and persistence of use were considered in both of the patient portal studies, but not addressed in the study design.

Digital Tools for Use Outside Clinical Settings that Communicates with the Electronic Health Record (Tele)

Digital tools that communicate with the EHR include tele solutions that enable patients to generate important data outside of the hospital or clinic setting as often as needed.

REMORA (REmote MOnitoring of Rheumatoid Arthritis) examines whether electronic collection of PROs directly from patients daily between clinic visits can enhance clinical care.[14] The "beta app" was tested by 8 patients for 1 month during which they completed routine questionnaires at home, with the data integrated into the EHR. Question sets included 7 visual analogue scales for daily symptoms including pain and fatigue; weekly self-reported counts of tender and swollen joints, flares, and impact on work; and monthly completion of the health assessment questionnaire (HAQ).[15] Patients were told that patient-generated health data would only be reviewed in clinic at the time of the encounter. Both patients and providers reported that the app and graphed results improved clinical care, made the consultation more personal, and demonstrated gradual improvements in symptoms in response to treatment that may otherwise have been missed, thereby supporting decision making. The app was therefore well received among a small, enthusiastic group of patients and providers, but future studies must determine feasibility of large-scale implementation and real impact on patient outcomes.

Salaffi and colleagues[16] showed that a scheduled intensive strategy, based on a tele monitoring system, was a useful approach to achieve remission after 1 year in 44 early patients with RA. Their telemedical tool, "RETE-MARCHE" included a Web site platform that patients accessed from their personal device to answer questions related to RA Impact of Disease (RAID). Importantly, the system immediately generated warnings to both the patient and the clinician case manager whenever it detected that the patient's self-monitoring showed deterioration in one or more of the symptoms monitored with RAID, in contrast to the REMORA study in which data were reviewed only at the next clinic visit with the provider. A higher percentage of patients in the telemonitoring group achieved Clinical Disease Activity Index (CDAI) remission versus patients managed conventionally (38.1% vs 25% at year 1, $P<.01$), and time to achieve remission was significantly shorter in the active group. In addition, the investigators determined the degree of patients' acceptance of the telemonitoring platform. An overall average of 4.28 on a scale of 5 indicated high patient satisfaction with the system. Furthermore, 90.5% said that they would keep using the system in the future. However, the study lacked information about clinicians' attitudes toward using the system, and the sample size of patients was small.

Finally, one study also described experiences with implementing a telePRO system, AmbuFlex, as the basis for follow-up in malignant and chronic diseases, including RA.[17] The patients defined the need for an outpatient consultation by delivering PROs using an online or paper questionnaire. The results were visually summarized and accessible via a link from the EHR, and the PROs were used to decide whether a patient needed an outpatient visit, based on an automated decision algorithm and published cutoff values. A total of 300 patients with RA from 2 outpatient clinics were referred to telePRO follow-up with an initial response rate to the questionnaire of 93% among these patients. No data were shown separately for patients with RA about how many of the incoming PRO questionnaires that could be handled with no further contact to the clinic than the PRO.

ELECTRONIC COLLECTION OF PATIENT-REPORTED OUTCOMES AT NATIONAL HEALTH SYSTEM LEVEL

As seen from the previous examples of digital tools, patient data are typically collected in a plethora of ways in individual health systems. There are, however, examples of nationwide efforts to reduce the heterogeneity in the types of data collected. Collecting PRO data from the patient once in connection to a clinical encounter in a structured and standardized manner has potential to help rheumatologists to provide better patient-centered care, researchers to have access to more accurate and comprehensive datasets, and allows departments to meet quality measures and conduct audits.

One example of a national PRO collection effort is the Danish DANBIO register. It is a national clinical research register and a data source for rheumatologic diseases (RA, axial spondyloarthritis, and psoriatic arthritis) for monitoring clinical quality at the national, regional, and hospital levels.[18] Patients report their symptoms on a touchscreen computer in the waiting room before the clinical encounter, and the data are later supplemented with clinician-derived data. Core variables, such as diagnosis, year of diagnosis, age, and gender, are registered at the first visit to a specialized hospital department or specialized private practice. Data entered at later visits include PROs for disease activity, pain, fatigue, functional status, and physician-reported objective measures of disease activity, treatment, and C-reactive protein. For some patients, variables such as quality of life, sociodemographic factors, lifestyle, and comorbidity are also registered.

DANBIO has high nationwide coverage and completeness on key data variables, and reporting is mandatory by law for all patients with RA. In 2015, the DANBIO cohort comprised approximately 26,000 patients with RA, 3200 patients with axial spondyloarthritis, and 6200 patients with psoriatic arthritis. Digital data are summarized graphically and used to populate a scoreboard for shared decision making between clinicians and patients during the visit (**Fig. 2**). The system is not yet integrated with the EHR, but works as a stand-alone tool, accessible from a secure Web site. DANBIO also works as a quality registry, an audit and feedback tool, and provides secondary use of data for research while fulfilling its primary purpose of supporting clinical care.

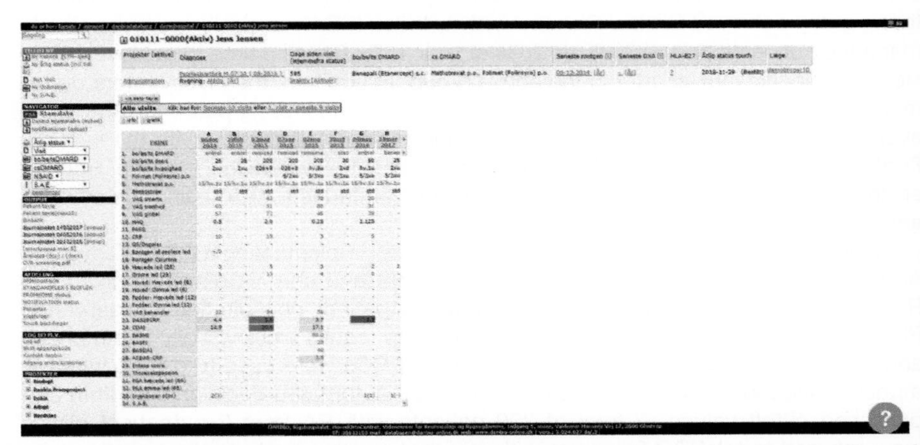

Fig. 2. Patient scoreboard in the Danish DANBIO register. The patient's disease is followed over time, and the scoreboard provides the physician and the patient with a comprehensive view of the treatment. Red: Severely active disease. Yellow: Moderately active disease. Green: Mildly active disease. (*Courtesy of* DANBIO, Denmark; with permission.)

No studies have yet been carried out to assess physicians' use of the DANBIO scoreboard to guide clinical decision making during patient visits.

Building a national infrastructure around the electronic collection of PRO data is also one of the aims of the American College of Rheumatology's RISE registry (Rheumatology Informatics System for Effectiveness). RISE passively extracts EHR data from participating practices, aggregates and analyzes the data centrally, and feeds this information back to clinicians as actionable data using a Web-based interface.[19] RISE is also a vehicle for quality reporting in the Merit-based Incentive Payment System (MIPS), a pay-for-performance program for physicians caring for Medicare beneficiaries. RISE currently houses one of the largest collections of outcomes among individuals with RA in the world, with almost half of 95,600 patients having an RA functional status assessment PRO measure and RA disease activity assessment in 2017.[20]

Unlike research performed within DANBIO, which is not integrated with a specific EHR, RISE has tackled the challenge of aggregating data from many different EHR systems that collect different measures during routine care. Although structured PRO data for patients with RA are available for many practices and collected via a diversity of methods (eg, paper, and then manually inputted into structured data fields in EHR note templates), some rheumatologists still record this information in the text of clinical notes. Therefore, RISE is working toward including critical information from unstructured fields like clinical notes by incorporating algorithms for text mining and natural language processing. These enhancements will increase the availability of PRO and other data for clinical research, performance measurement, and population health management at the individual practice level.

DISCUSSION

This review illustrates that current electronic PRO systems within EHRs and freestanding systems outside the EHR have varied significantly to date in their focus and features. PRO assessments have been incorporated into the clinic visit by several electronic means, and workflow considerations have been fundamental to the successful integration into care settings. Overall, well thought-out collection of electronic PROs has potential to bridge the gap between health care providers and patient perspectives in rheumatology by focusing the clinical encounter more on the individual patient's experience and perceptions of disease impact. We summarize the key lessons learned from the literature to date in the following sections.

Lesson 1: the Importance of Attention to Workflow

Studies of many of the previously mentioned health IT tools, whether fully integrated or stand-alone, raised concerns about workflow changes in clinical practice and patient engagement after implementation as barriers to adoption. Systematic ePRO collection and delivery to health care providers to use for clinical decision making will clearly not be fully embraced if it is perceived to disrupt or impede clinical workflow. This was exemplified by Li and colleagues,[13] in which one of the investigators' goals for online collection was to decrease the burden of data collection and data entry for the clinic staff. However, the workflow still required that medical assistants assessed whether a patient already completed PROs through the patient portal at the time of patient check-in, and this process was both time-consuming and error prone. Yen and colleagues[6] also received mixed feedback from clinicians toward their stand-alone PRO tool with concerns mainly questioning the implementation of a mobile application into the clinical workflow and how it may impact patient care.

One way to avoid the pitfall of negative or unintended consequences during implementation is to identify all stakeholders who are likely to be involved with the tool early in the development and engage these stakeholders in the design and testing process and ultimately in ongoing improvements. Participatory design, such as human-centered design thinking, deeply engages the end-user in the design process.[21] Similarly, process redesign methodologies, such as plan-do-study-act (PDSA), focus intensively on changing the workflows by small-scale rapid-cycle tests of change as a form of iterative "learning in action" to ensure that any modifiable obstacles to implementation are addressed.[22] Based on our review, few studies have used human-centered design thinking and few report systematic redesign or quality improvement methodologies. Attention to workflow considerations will reduce burden of collection, increase reliability of PRO capture, and reduce nonuse of results. For example, the most successful efforts to date, such as Rheum-PACER, undertook a rigorous workflow redesign process, with careful attention to physician and staff workload.[3]

Before building Rheum-PACER, Newman and colleagues[23] additionally explored how a computerized version of the MDHAQ (Multidimensional Health Assessment Questionnaire) could be adopted for routine use in a busy, complex, and resource-constrained rheumatology department. PDSA was used in 2 cycles of workflow redesign during implementation of a touchscreen questionnaire, and it was shown that the routine use of a touchscreen questionnaire can be tightly integrated with routine clinical care by focusing on continuous problem solving as well as design and workflow issues.

Our own experiences using a human-centered design process included patients, providers, and staff at 2 outpatient clinics, and evolved around the development of a PRO dashboard for patients with RA.[24] We conducted clinic observations, interviews with stakeholders, patient and provider focus groups, and iteratively prototyped and tested the dashboard in clinical settings in close collaboration with health IT designers. The result was a PRO-focused dashboard that supports a conversation about treatment, centered on the patient's most salient goals, concerns, and experiences, with the overall aim of facilitating shared decision making.

Although the process of designing the tool's user interface and the selection of PROs included in the tools are infrequently discussed,[25,26] these are critical steps in the development of successful digital tools.[4] This ensures that the integration happens in a way that meets the needs of the various users, and may support relevance and appropriateness with the goal to reduce nonresponse or sluggish uptake.

Lesson 2: Integration into the Health Information Technology Ecosystem

Increasingly, workflow redesign requires consideration of the health IT ecosystem, including the capabilities of EHR systems and the capacity of those systems for data integration. This has been a significant barrier for many efforts, and there is a clear lack of interoperability between systems, without the possibility of easily customizing data flow into EHRs. As an example, despite being designed for quality and research purposes and as a point of care tool to aid in clinical decision making, the DANBIO register is still, almost 20 years after go-live, not integrated into hospital EHRs due to interoperability issues between IT systems and different EHR vendors.

As evidenced by the tools reviewed here, success with EHR integration has varied significantly. To be useful, PRO data should be easy to interpret and actionable.[23] Integrating electronic PRO data directly into the EHR ensures that clinicians get the right information at the right time (during the encounter) and allows tracking over time in relation to other clinical information available in the EHR (eg, laboratory tests and medication). In contrast, incorporating stand-alone applications into the clinic visit often requires that the physician exit the EHR to retrieve and view data. Alternatively, clinic staff can manually enter data such as calculated disease activity scores from the stand-alone application into the EHR, again adding an extra manual task to the workflow.[27] Stand-alone tools, on the other hand, are often less expensive, and provide a good opportunity to test if an electronic capture system works for patients and providers in practice, or to assess the validity of new ePROs against their paper counterparts as seen in several of our included studies.[7] Some EHR vendors, including Epic and Cerner systems, are creating systems and interfaces that allow outside applications to be supported and integrated with their software, although successful demonstration projects in rheumatology are still lacking, and interfaces to write to the EHR (rather than merely support read-only access) has been elusive.

Lesson 3: Minimize Patient Burden

From the patient's point of view, minimizing data collection burden is essential and fatigability of use is important. Features enabled by online EHR patient portals offer a platform to further coordinate and develop PRO collection beyond the clinical encounter, further enhancing patient PRO monitoring.[28]

Li and colleagues[13] found that even though most of their included patients had an active online portal account, only a fraction (fewer than 20%) completed the patient portal PROMIS survey before an in-person visit. Uptake of portals was found in a systematic review to differ by patient-specific factors with lower use by racial and ethnic minorities and lower use with lower education level or literacy,[28] and this was furthermore echoed by Li and colleagues.[13] More widespread acceptance will require attention to overcoming these barriers and addressing usability and patient-perceived value to engage certain populations. This might include providing materials about enrollment, tools, and surveys in multiple languages and for patients with low literacy. In addition, more work is required to ensure that collected data are useful to patients and meaningfully impacts factors such as their ability to monitor and manage their condition and communicate with their physician. Future studies should address issues of portal access, enrollment, satisfaction, and persistence to accommodate the needs and preferences of diverse populations.

Lesson 4: What Happens Between Visits Matters

Technology, such as smartphone apps, enables patients to generate important data outside of the hospital setting as often as needed and share it with their providers to expand the depth, breadth, and continuity of information available.[29] Digital tools relying on these tele-strategies allow PRO data capture between visits, and provide a more accurate and quantifiable representation of disease activity that can be incorporated into clinical decision making as seen with REMORA.[14] Rather than relying on retrospective patient recall at clinic encounters, with its inherent biases, remote collection of PROs can help develop a clear picture of symptoms over time and highlight areas of importance that might be missed when relying on patients' subsequent recall during the consultation.[30] Patients care about what happens between visits, and feel that reporting between hospital or clinic visits better reflects their health. Patients using the REMORA app reported that the app made care "more personal to you" and "found it made a difference, because it wasn't all me telling him and trying to remember. The information was there so you've got solid proof straightaway."[15] This feedback suggests that the data recorded remotely between visits matters, and that it most likely will have a number of benefits for both patients and clinicians.

This functionality, though, presents challenges, such as reaching and engaging patients without Internet access at home and determining the appropriate clinical response (if any) for PRO scores that indicate problems warranting immediate clinical attention. This is particularly true because physicians currently express that data review burden in clinical practice is already high, even without data collected outside the clinical setting. Finally, strict attention to the accuracy of clinical decision support that recommends a clinical response should be given, to ensure that safety in relation to detecting patients in need of attention is not compromised.[17]

Lesson 5: Pragmatic Study Designs

Despite the significant enthusiasm about digital tools in clinical practice, rigorously tested tools that clearly improve patient outcomes are scant. Internally, the use of evaluation and quality improvement techniques can be used to illustrate how PRO implementation adds value in a clinical encounter. Demonstrating value to a broader audience requires additional outcomes, including the user experience (patient and provider attitudes, satisfaction with the system, doctor-patient communication), health services outcomes (clinical actions taken, referrals), and patient outcomes.[31]

A recent editorial from *The Lancet* pointed out that "*continuing to argue for digital exceptionalism and failing to robustly evaluate digital health interventions presents the greatest risk for patients and health systems.*"[32] Randomized controlled trials, the gold standard of evidence, are rarely used in evaluation of digital health interventions and are often challenging to fund; only one of the rheumatology-specific tools we included underwent this sort of rigorous testing. This might be due in part to the costs of conducting such a trial, which are high relative to the tools' perceived very low level of risk for the patient. Randomized controlled trials also can be difficult in the experimental evaluation of these tools because of cost, time, and difficulty (including acceptability) in randomizing different providers or health systems to the health IT intervention.

However, rheumatology still needs to build an evidence base showing which strategies are most successful in improving patient outcomes, minimizing adverse events, and maximizing patient as well as provider satisfaction. Quasi-experimental or pragmatic study designs without randomization might be one way to thoroughly evaluate digital interventions. Such studies compare an outcome of interest by using pre- and postintervention measurement of the same measure, and have been shown to be useful when evaluating new health system interventions.[33]

SUMMARY

Technology exists that can foster understanding the patients' experience of their illness in a way that was previously not possible. Early experience in using technology to capture this information through PROs within the field of rheumatology suggests that careful attention to human-centered design, including detailed workflow planning, consideration of patient and physician burden, integration into the health IT ecosystem, and delivering information to the right person at the right time to ensure it is actionable are important. For PRO collection to have a meaningful impact on patient outcomes, all of the previously described considerations need to be woven into the design of applications, and importantly, they must be tested in diverse health systems and in diverse populations, including diseases other than RA, to ensure they are simple to interpret, useful for clinical decision making, and effective in impacting outcomes.

REFERENCES

1. Dixon WG, Michaud K. Using technology to support clinical care and research in rheumatoid arthritis. Curr Opin Rheumatol 2018;30(3):276–81.

2. Callahan LF. The history of patient-reported outcomes in rheumatology. Rheum Dis Clin North Am 2016;42(2):205–17.
3. Newman ED, Lerch V, Billet J, et al. Improving the quality of care of patients with rheumatic disease using patient-centric electronic redesign software. Arthritis Care Res (Hoboken) 2015;67(4):546–53.
4. Schmajuk G, Yazdany J. Leveraging the electronic health record to improve quality and safety in rheumatology. Rheumatol Int 2017;37(10):1603–10.
5. US Food and Drug Administration. Guidance for industry: patient-reported outcome measures: use in medical product development to support labeling claims: draft guidance. Health Qual Life Outcomes 2006;4:79.
6. Yen PY, Lara B, Lopetegui M, et al. Usability and workflow evaluation of "RhEumAtic Disease activitY" (READY). A mobile application for rheumatology patients and providers. Appl Clin Inform 2016;7(4):1007–24.
7. El Miedany Y, El Gaafary M, Youssef S, et al. Toward electronic health recording: evaluation of electronic patient-reported outcome measures system for remote monitoring of early rheumatoid arthritis. J Rheumatol 2016;43(12):2106–12.
8. Salaffi F, Gasparini S, Ciapetti A, et al. Usability of an innovative and interactive electronic system for collection of patient-reported data in axial spondyloarthritis: comparison with the traditional paper-administered format. Rheumatology (Oxford) 2013;52(11):2062–70.
9. Coons SJ, Gwaltney CJ, Hays RD, et al. Recommendations on evidence needed to support measurement equivalence between electronic and paper-based patient-reported outcome (PRO) measures: ISPOR ePRO Good Research Practices Task Force report. Value Health 2009;12(4):419–29.
10. Collier DS, Kay J, Estey G, et al. A rheumatology-specific informatics-based application with a disease activity calculator. Arthritis Rheum 2009;61(4):488–94.
11. Chua RM, Mecchella JN, Zbehlik AJ. Improving the measurement of disease activity for patients with rheumatoid arthritis: validation of an electronic version of the routine assessment of patient index data 3. Int J Rheumatol 2015;2015:834070.
12. Epis OM, Casu C, Belloli L, et al. Pixel or paper? Validation of a mobile technology for collecting patient-reported outcomes in rheumatoid arthritis. JMIR Res Protoc 2016;5(4):e219.
13. Li J, Yazdany J, Trupin L, et al. Capturing a patient-reported measure of physical function through an online electronic health record patient portal in an ambulatory clinic: implementation study. JMIR Med Inform 2018;6(2):e31.
14. Dixon WG, Sanders C, Austin L. Identifying key variables for inclusion in a smartphone app to support clinical care and research in patients with rheumatoid arthritis. 2016. Available at: https://acrabstracts.org/abstract/identifying-key-variables-for-inclusion-in-a-smartphone-app-to-support-clinical-care-and-research-in-patients-with-rheumatoid-arthritis/. Accessed September 3, 2018.
15. Austin L, Sanders C, Dixon WG. Patients' experiences of using a smartphone app for remote monitoring of rheumatoid arthritis, integrated into the electronic medical record, and its impact on consultations. 2016. Available at: https://acrabstracts.org/abstract/patients-experiences-of-using-a-smartphone-app-for-remote-monitoring-of-rheumatoid-arthritis-integrated-into-the-electronic-medical-record-and-its-impact-on-consultations/. Accessed September 3, 2016.
16. Salaffi F, Carotti M, Ciapetti A, et al. Effectiveness of a telemonitoring intensive strategy in early rheumatoid arthritis: comparison with the conventional management approach. BMC Musculoskelet Disord 2016;17:146.

17. Schougaard LM, Larsen LP, Jessen A, et al. AmbuFlex: tele-patient-reported outcomes (telePRO) as the basis for follow-up in chronic and malignant diseases. Qual Life Res 2016;25(3):525–34.
18. Ibfelt EH, Jensen DV, Hetland ML. The Danish nationwide clinical register for patients with rheumatoid arthritis: DANBIO. Clin Epidemiol 2016;8:737–42.
19. Yazdany J, Bansback N, Clowse M, et al. Rheumatology informatics system for effectiveness: a national informatics-enabled registry for quality improvement. Arthritis Care Res (Hoboken) 2016;68(12):1866–73.
20. Yazdany J, Johansson T, Myslinski R, et al. Performance on quality measures in the RISE registry and the merit-based incentive payment system (MIPS). 2017;69(suppl 10). Available at: https://acrabstracts.org/abstract/performance-on-quality-measures-in-the-rise-registry-and-the-merit-based-incentive-payment-system-mips/. Accessed October 28, 2018.
21. Johnson CM, Johnson TR, Zhang J. A user-centered framework for redesigning health care interfaces. J Biomed Inform 2005;38(1):75–87.
22. Taylor MJ, McNicholas C, Nicolay C, et al. Systematic review of the application of the plan-do-study-act method to improve quality in healthcare. BMJ Qual Saf 2014;23(4):290–8.
23. Newman ED, Lerch V, Jones JB, et al. Touchscreen questionnaire patient data collection in rheumatology practice: development of a highly successful system using process redesign. Arthritis Care Res (Hoboken) 2012;64(4):589–96.
24. Ragouzeos D, Gandrup J, Berrean B, et al. "Am I OK?" Using human centered design to empower rheumatoid arthritis patients through patient reported outcomes. Patient Educ Couns 2018. [Epub ahead of print].
25. Schick-Makaroff K, Molzahn A. Strategies to use tablet computers for collection of electronic patient-reported outcomes. Health Qual Life Outcomes 2015;13:2.
26. El Miedany Y, El Gaafary M, El Aroussy N, et al. Toward electronic health recording: evaluation of electronic patient reported outcome measures (e-PROMs) system for remote monitoring of early systemic lupus patients. Clin Rheumatol 2017;36(11):2461–9.
27. Bays A, Wahl E, Daikh DI, et al. Implementation of disease activity measurement for rheumatoid arthritis patients in an academic rheumatology clinic. BMC Health Serv Res 2016;16(a):384.
28. Goldzweig CL, Orshansky G, Paige NM, et al. Electronic patient portals: evidence on health outcomes, satisfaction, efficiency, and attitudes: a systematic review. Ann Intern Med 2013;159(10):677–87.
29. Deering MJ. Issue brief: patient-generated health data and health IT 2013. Available at: https://www.healthit.gov/topic/scientific-initiatives/patient-generated-health-data. Accessed September 29, 2018.
30. Piga M, Cangemi I, Mathieu A, et al. Telemedicine for patients with rheumatic diseases: systematic review and proposal for research agenda. Semin Arthritis Rheum 2017;47(1):121–8.
31. Jensen RE, Rothrock NE, DeWitt EM, et al. The role of technical advances in the adoption and integration of patient-reported outcomes in clinical care. Med Care 2015;53(2):153–9.
32. The Lancet. Is digital medicine different? Lancet 2018;392(10142):95.
33. Ramsay CR, Matowe L, Grilli R, et al. Interrupted time series designs in health technology assessment: lessons from two systematic reviews of behavior change strategies. Int J Technol Assess Health Care 2003;19(4):613–23.

APPENDIX 1: STRUCTURED REVIEW

We performed a structured review of the literature to assess the nature and extent of current digital tools being used to collect PROs in clinical rheumatology settings. Specifically, we focused on the design; implementation strategies; EHR integration status; whether clinics, providers, and patients adopted the new form of administration; and how it impacted clinic workflow. In addition, we focused on evaluation of patient outcomes, time to document, and satisfaction as measures of effectiveness.

With the assistance of a professional librarian, we searched 2 electronic databases (PubMed and EmBase), from August 2018 and 10 years back; MeSH terms and search concepts are listed in **Table 2**. We evaluated gray literature, including proceedings from major rheumatology meetings (American College of Rheumatology [ACR] and the European League Against Rheumatism from 2008 to 2018), and conducted hand searches of reference lists of retrieved articles.

Studies evaluating use of PROs in a clinical trial or in a pediatric setting were excluded, as were articles describing use of PROs in evaluating orthopedic management of musculoskeletal conditions such as total joint arthroplasty for osteoarthritis. Studies on applications that allow patients to track symptoms and self-manage their disease without involvement of the clinic or clinician were also excluded.

We identified 192 titles by the search, and following screening of titles and abstracts, 10 tools were included in this review. One additional tool was identified by screening the ACR abstract archive. Nine of 10 studies targeted patients with RA and their providers. Patient and provider satisfaction was the most common outcome among the included studies. Validation of electronic collection of validated PRO questionnaires against their traditional paper counterparts were reported by 5 studies. Design, workflow changes, and adoption were less frequently mentioned. Explicit discussions of whether this strategy led to improvements in patient outcomes, were rarely included, demonstrating the need for guidance on how to best evaluate tools to maximize their use.

Table 2
MeSH terms used for structured review of digital tools to collect PRO

Search Concepts	Search Terms
1. Patient-reported outcomes	((((“Patient-Reported Outcome” OR “Patient-Reported Outcomes” OR “Patient Reported Outcomes” OR “Patient Reported Outcome” OR “Patient Reported Outcome Measure”[MeSH] OR “Patient Reported Outcome Measures” OR “PROMs” OR “PROMIS” OR “PRO-PM” OR “e-PROM” OR “e-PROMS” OR “Self Report”[MeSH] OR “Disease Activity”))
2. Digital tools	((("Mobile Applications"[Mesh] OR mhealth OR m-health OR “mobile health” OR “health IT” OR “health information technology” OR digital OR ipad OR “mobile apps” OR “Smartphone” OR “EHR” OR “electronic health record” OR “electronic health records” OR “mobile device” OR “mobile devices” OR “EMR” OR “electronic medical record” OR “electronic medical records” OR “patient portal” OR "Patient Portals"[Mesh] OR “Electronic assessment”)))
3. Diseases	((("Rheumatic Diseases"[Mesh] OR "rheumatoid arthritis" OR "arthritis, rheumatoid"[mesh] OR rheumatology OR rheumatologic OR rheumatologist OR rheumatologists OR Spondylarthropathies [MeSH] OR “Lupus Erythematosus, Systemic” [MeSH] OR “Scleroderma, Systemic” [MeSH] OR “Vasculitis” [MeSH] OR “Myositis”[MeSH] OR “Mixed connective tissue disease” [MeSH] OR “rheumatic disease” OR “rheumatic diseases” OR “rheumatoid arthritis” OR lupus OR scleroderma OR vasculitis OR myositis OR “ankylosing spondylitis” OR “psoriatic arthritis” OR “reactive arthritis”)))

Tools and Methods for Real-World Evidence Generation

Pragmatic Trials, Electronic Consent, and Data Linkages

Jeffrey R. Curtis, MD, MS, MPH*, P. Jeff Foster, MPH, Kenneth G. Saag, MD, MSc

KEYWORDS

- Pragmatic trials • Real-world evidence • Rheumatoid arthritis • Osteoporosis
- Data linkage • Informed consent

KEY POINTS

- Efficient generation of real-world evidence demands new tools to answer questions of high importance to patients, clinicians, researchers, policymakers, and other stakeholders.
- Pragmatic trials that study well-defined outcomes in highly generalizable patient populations can provide direct evidence about risks and benefits of medical interventions.
- Technology-based tools (eg, apps running on mobile devices) that facilitate electronic consent for research participation can effectively enable efficient screening and recruitment for pragmatic trials and real-world studies.
- New methods for linkages between disparate data sources can enrich the types of information available for research purposes and can accommodate a wide spectrum of constraints around the nature and extent of the identifiable information that can be shared.

INTRODUCTION

Real-world evidence (RWE) on clinical effectiveness has assumed increasingly greater importance over time in the practice of medicine. Given the recognition that a majority of what is done in clinical practice is not supported by direct evidence, clinicians,

Disclosures: None.
This work was supported by NIAMS UM1 AR065705, NIAMS 1R21AR062300, 1U34AR062891, and PCORI PRN-1306-04811A02.
Division of Clinical Immunology and Rheumatology, University of Alabama at Birmingham, Birmingham, AL, USA
* Corresponding author. 510 20th Street South, Faculty Office Towers 802, Birmingham, AL 35294.
E-mail address: jcurtis@uab.edu

Rheum Dis Clin N Am 45 (2019) 275–289
https://doi.org/10.1016/j.rdc.2019.01.010
rheumatic.theclinics.com

researchers, policy makers, regulatory agencies, and other stakeholders are turning their attention to evidence that has better generalizability to inform the practical decisions that they must make day to day. Real-world data that are used for evidence generation often refer to information about health care derived from multiple sources that are outside the typical confines of research (eg, randomized controlled trials [RCTs] of highly selected individuals).[1]

The hoped-for benefits of generating evidence and obtaining it from routine care settings, as may be recorded in electronic medical record (EMR) systems, administrative claims data (eg, pharmacy refill data), mobile health, and other diverse sources, is not only to improve the generalizability of research but also to expand the available evidence for patients with significant disease heterogeneity, multimorbidity, and more severe disease manifestations than typically permitted in an RCT. For example, the proportion of rheumatoid arthritis (RA) patients seen in routine care settings who would be eligible for a typical phase 3 RCT has been estimated to be 20% or even lower.[2,3] Additional factors that may affect clinical outcomes that would be irrelevant, or considered nuisance factors in an RCT, can also be studied more effectively using real-world data. For example, aspects of the health care delivery system, clinician-related and provider-related factors (eg, primary care vs specialty providers), and patient-related influences, including infrastructure (eg, local care pathways and treatment patterns, and on-site infusion capabilities), accessibility (eg, distance to clinical site and appointment wait times), socioeconomic status, specific comorbidities, and medication adherence, all can affect outcomes. These can be studied as components of RWE generation and thus improve the generalizability of research findings.

A common misconception is that RWE requires researchers to stay firmly grounded in the demesne of observational studies. RWE, however, is compatible with the ability to randomize and deliver an intervention, if that is needed. Randomization can be at the individual patient level or at a group or site level (eg, cluster randomization),[4] which may facilitate practical study implementation and help avoid confounding related to inadvertent provider-specific or site-specific influences on the study intervention that might apply to all patients treated at that site. The 21st Century Cures Act enabled the Food and Drug Administration (FDA) to include RWE in the regulatory process, which may encompass activities, including drug label expansions and postmarketing surveillance programs.[5] For all these reasons and more, RWE presents an unprecedented opportunity to extend the research enterprise beyond the typical bounds of academia and to optimally create a true learning health care system whereby research is seamlessly integrated into clinical care. To do so effectively, however, will require new tools and approaches for evidence generation. This article is informed by exemplar case studies in rheumatology, with a focus on the design features of an RCT of the live zoster vaccine in biologic-treated patients that illustrate use of new tools and methods, including pragmatic trials, electronic patient consent, and data linkages.

PRAGMATIC TRIALS

Explanatory Versus Pragmatic Trials

Historically, most clinical RCTs have been explanatory in nature. The focus of such trials is efficacy, that is, whether the intervention (eg, drug, treatment strategy, or medical procedure) works under ideal conditions. These studies, aimed at confirming that the desired therapeutics work as well in humans as early studies in vitro and in animals might suggest, are critical for regularly approval of drugs, devices, and biologics. Patients tend to be highly selected, however, and those with any anticipated impediments to full adherence to the study protocol are excluded at the outset. The study is monitored closely for adherence to the protocol, and endpoints may be biologic proxies for the outcome (eg, changes in a biomarker or laboratory test) or process measures (eg, delivery of care or a specified clinical action taken, at the prescribed time). Often, however, these trials can only provide indirect evidence for clinicians, patients, and policymakers who need these data to make decisions. In contrast, pragmatic trials focus on effectiveness (ie, Does the intervention work in normal practice?). Inclusion criteria in pragmatic trials are often less restrictive, and an all-comers approach that is representative of the patients seen in real-world settings is preferred. Optimally, the investigators should be closer to routine practitioners and less likely to be large research shops where many phase 3 studies are conducted. Interventions are applied as they would be in routine clinical care, and, as such, these trials are intended to generate direct evidence about the population to which the intervention will be ultimately applied. In contrast to explanatory studies, these studies typically trade off better generalizability for lower internal validity. Features of explanatory versus pragmatic trials have been summarized[6] and described along a continuum known as the pragmatic-explanatory continuum indicatory summary[7] (**Fig. 1**).

Features that facilitate the conduct of a pragmatic trial include study outcomes that are simpler and more objectively defined (eg, a discrete event such as a well-defined

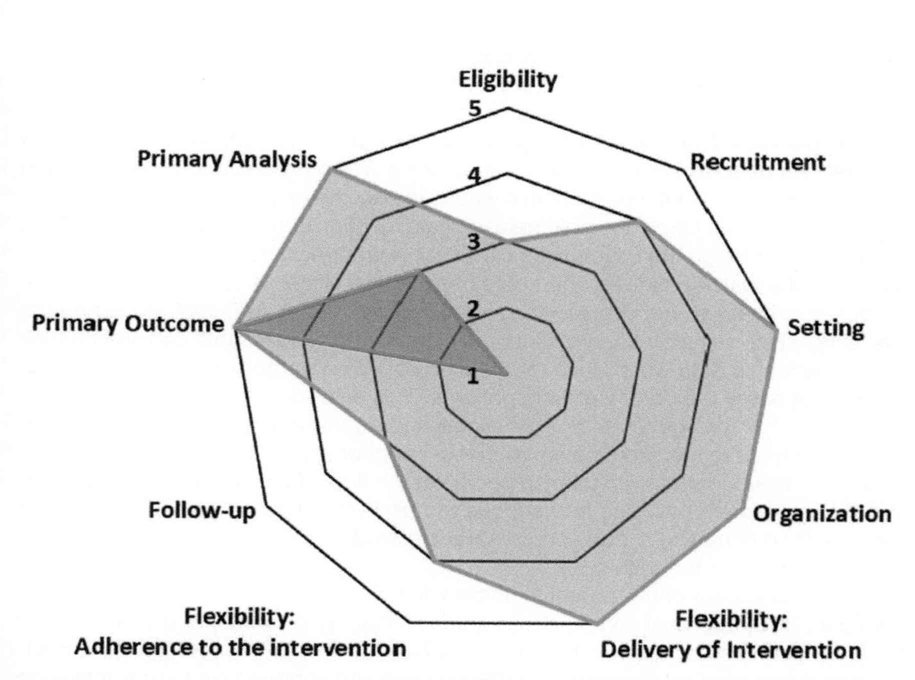

Fig. 1. PRECIS-2 Wheel Illustrating Continuum between Pragmatic and Explanatory Trials using Two Osteoporosis Trial Examples. Note: Trials that are more pragmatic generate a wheel with its circumference closer to the rim and have a higher rank on the PRECIS 5 point Likert scale; those that are more explanatory are closer to the hub.[7] Figure based on study design of the Effectiveness of DiscontinuinG bisphosphonatEs (EDGE, blue shading)[20] and The Fracture Intervention Trial Long Term Extension (FLEX, orange shading) trials.[43]

infection, fracture, myocardial infarction, or death), an intervention that can be delivered efficiently in a relatively simple fashion, and a pool of motivated participants (including both patients and providers) who are willing to participate.

A Practical Example: The VaricEcella zosteR VaccinE Trial

Although a variety of pragmatic trials have been conducted in medicine[8–10] and in rheumatology,[11] the design features of the VaricEcella zosteR VaccinE (VERVE) trial illustrate many of the relevant concepts of a pragmatic trial.[12] VERVE is a blinded RCT of patients aged 50 and older receiving anti–tumor necrosis factor (TNF) therapy who are randomized to receive the live zoster vaccine or placebo (saline). VERVE has simple inclusion criteria, and, unless someone is being actively treated for malignancy, has a meaningful other source of immunosuppression (eg, transplant or high-dose glucocorticoid use), previously received the live zoster vaccine, or could become pregnant, all patients on any of the 5 TNF inhibitor therapies are eligible to participate. There are no disease-specific requirements (eg, RA, psoriasis, or inflammatory bowel disease), and even off-label use of TNF inhibitor treatment is permitted (eg, sarcoidosis). A key motivating concern that has tempered enthusiasm to use this attenuated, live virus vaccine for patients receiving biologic treatments is the potential for the vaccine to cause a weakened form of the very infection (ie, varicella zoster, manifested as chicken pox) that it is intended to reduce complications for. For that reason, safety is a main outcome of the study.

If patients were to develop vaccine-strain varicella infection related to the vaccine, it is expected to occur early (eg, within 4 weeks). Therefore, VERVE has its second and only follow-up visit at week 6 (to allow for a comfortable margin past 4 weeks). At this visit, as at the baseline visit, biospecimens are collected for the trial to assess the trials' immunologic-based outcomes (eg, glycoprotein ELISA and changes in cytokines measured via peripheral blood mononuclear cells). Were a patient to develop a rash suggestive of varicella infection within 6 weeks of vaccine (or placebo) administration, skin swabs would be taken and polymerase chain reaction performed to verify varicella infection, and subtype the infection as either vaccine-strain versus wild-type strain.

Because the trial needed large numbers of patients to meet its objectives (eg, >600), an efficient process to both screen for and recruit patients is essential. Based on the trials' simply inclusion criteria, providers and health care systems that can search their EMR or electronic data warehouse for patients based on demographics and medication use can easily preidentify eligible patients. This electronic screening using tools, such as i2b2,[13,14] can generate a list of eligible individuals and enable a study coordinator to reach out to them (eg, patient portal or telephone) prior to their next upcoming visit and/or make contact with them in person at the time of their next routine appointment. This approach provides tremendous recruitment efficiency compared with the typical method of having a study coordinator passively wait for a clinician to refer patients individually to the trial.

As one final aspect of the potential efficiencies of a pragmatic trial, institutional review board (IRB) approval can be streamlined. A majority (23 of 33) of the VERVE trial sites were governed by a single IRB. The new National Institutes of Health (NIH) guidance that is intended to streamline the IRB process and shorten time to trial activation will require that even multisite trials use only a single IRB for approval.[15] The Streamlined, Multisite, Accelerated Resources for Trials (SMART) IRB platform provides a flexible, efficient enhanced version that extends capacities previously served by traditional reliance agreements, whereby only 1 IRB governs the conduct of the study, and all other sites (including academic medical centers) rely on the single, central IRB for oversight. Both academic medical centers and commercial IRBs (eg, Advarra and Western IRB) can serve to provide oversight for SMART IRB–approved studies.

ELECTRONIC SCREENING AND CONSENT

A variety of barriers exist to a general clinician's participation in pragmatic clinical trials.[16–19] As one of those barriers, the time commitment and feasibility of not only screening for eligible patients but also facilitating the process of obtaining informed consent from a patient can be burdensome in a busy clinical setting not routinely devoted to clinical trials. The details of the trial must be explained to patients in a clear fashion, and specific elements of the study as described in the informed consent document approved by an IRB must be presented. Although the IRBs can provide well-defined guidance about what an informed consent document must contain and undergoes careful scrutiny by the IRB itself, the often informal information provided regarding the study's nature, objectives, and details may be highly variable when communicated by a study investigator or research coordinator to a patient. To reduce variability in the understanding of the VERVE trial's key elements, a tablet-based (iPad) interactive system was developed and deployed to explain the study and facilitate obtaining informed consent. Potential participants are asked a series of short questions related to the trial's few inclusion criteria (eg, current use of any of the give anti-TNF therapies, current treatment of malignancy, cessation of menstruation for more than a year [to avoid enrolling women who might become pregnant], and prior receipt of the zoster vaccine) to affirm eligibility. Patients are then presented a custom 6-minute to 7-minute video (**Fig. 2**) developed specifically for the study that explains its details in clear and simple terms. The study coordinator (who in a Pragmatic Clinical Trial (PCT) may be a clinic staff person less well versed in research) need not be even in the room as the video is viewed.

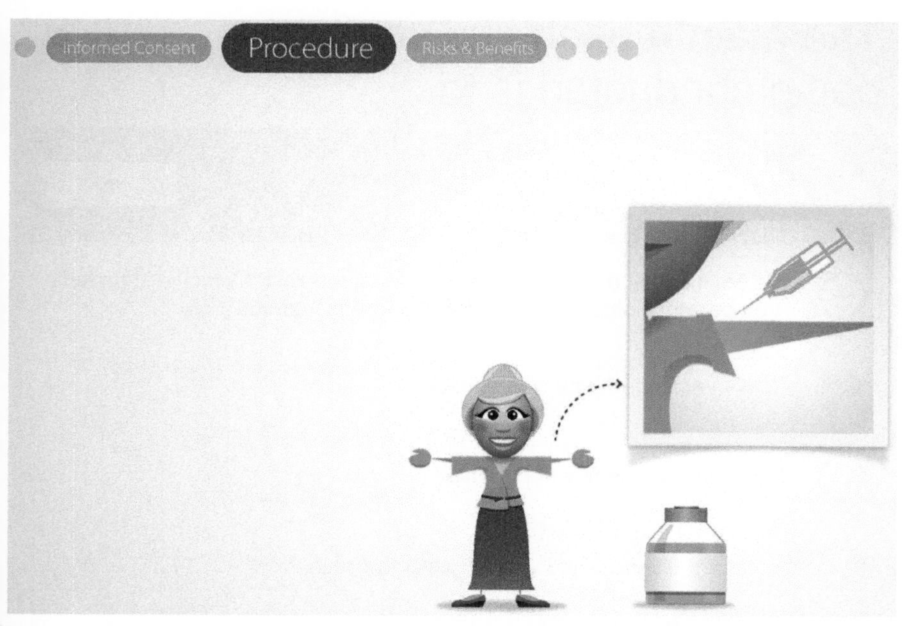

Fig. 2. Example of iPad tablet–based study video describing the VERVE pragmatic trial.

After the patient has watched the required video, the informed consent document is presented on the tablet, and the patient can depress the screen to obtain more information and pop up a dictionary definition for any of the specific terms mentioned in the consent document. Having read the consent document, the patient is asked a series of questions to confirm that the essential elements of the trial are understood. If a patient does not answer correctly, and assuming the consenting clinicians believe obtaining true informed consent for this patient is indeed possible, the knowledge gap can sometimes be remediated, and the potential participant hyperlinked back to the relevant section of the informed consent document to refer back to the appropriate information in the informed consent document (**Fig. 3**). Having pilot tested this assessment process during the development of a different pragmatic trial focused on bisphosphonate drug holidays,[20] a focus group of IRB members as well as the IRBs governing the VERVE trial generally found it highly acceptable, particularly compared with the typical requirement that is generally satisfied (from a documentation standpoint) by a patient's initials appearing on the bottom of every page of the informed consent and their signature at the end. The consent process can also entail any number of revisions or customizations required by a local IRB or by state and local regulations. For example, the state of California has specific requirements for research participation,[21,22] including the requirement to present to potential patients the text of the "Experimental Research Subject's Bill of Rights," which was made available on the tablet to the California participants considering the trial. Finally, patients are

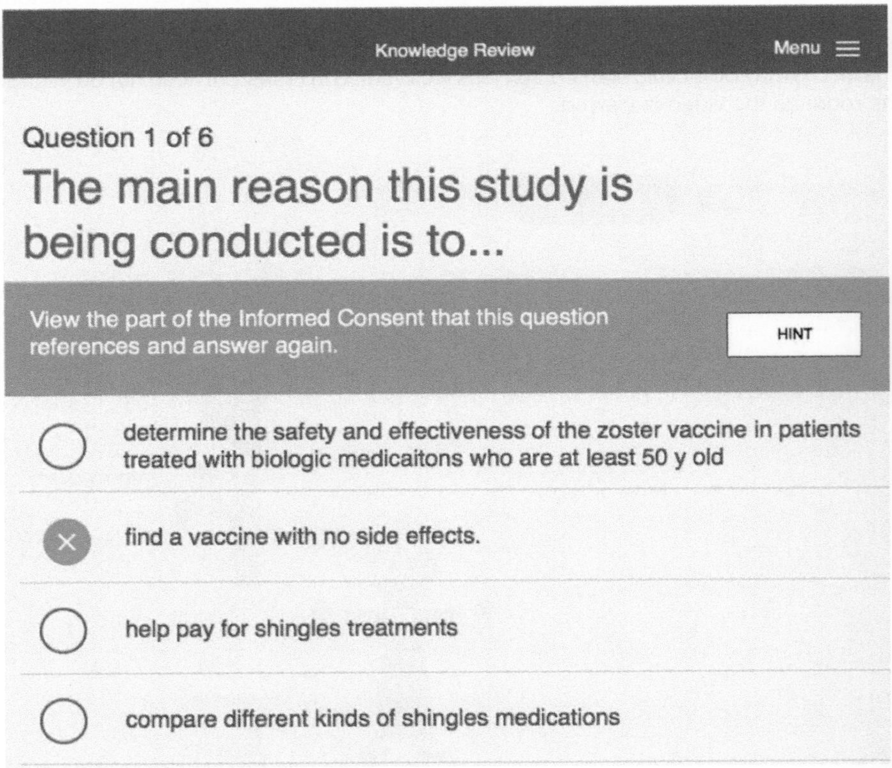

Fig. 3. Assessing patients' understanding of the VERVE pragmatic trial deployed on a tablet.

afforded the opportunity to ask questions of the research coordinator and site investigator, who provide an electronic countersignature to confirm enrollment.

Overall, the process of using a tablet computer to obtain informed consent from patients for a pragmatic trial was found highly acceptable based on experience from a pilot study,[23] and site staff and patients generally preferred, or were at least as comfortable with, the tablet-based method compared with its traditional paper equivalent. In the conduct of the VERVE trial, and based on 613 patients randomized through November 2018, 7.9% of patients who initiated the electronic consent process (and presumably had been deemed tentatively eligible for the study) answered the screening questions in a way that precluded their participation, and only 13% of people who started the electronic consent process elected to not participate. Overall, the electronic consent process was deemed acceptable and feasible by VERVE trial sites, although 1 of the 33 VERVE trial sites initially was not permitted by the local IRB to participate because consent was obtained electronically. The site later reversed its position, perhaps facilitated by the eConsent guidance from the FDA and the Department of Health and Human Services that was carefully adopted for the VERVE trial.[24]

Once patients decide to participate, their signature is collected electronically on the tablet (ie, with their finger or stylus). This feature, coupled with the few patient-facing screening questions and short data collection elements, are deployed on the tablet, obviating need for paper case report forms filled out by patients that must be manually entered by a study coordinator into the trials' electronic data capture system. Instead, a messaging service between the tablet's centralized and cloud-based database transmits the information directly to the electronic data capture system (which, in VERVE, is hosted by another vendor). Additional aspects to the electronic capture of a patient's signature also enables efficient capture of the patient's permission for two additional important elements of the study authorization, a Health Insurance Portability and Accountability Act of 1996 (HIPAA) authorization and a medical record release form, used for purposes discussed later. As 1 final feature of the study that was facilitated by use of the tablet-based system, if a patient presents within the 6 weeks after receipt of the zoster vaccine (or placebo) with a rash that might be varicella infection (or, less likely, shingles reactivation), the camera on the iPad is used to take one or more photographs of the rash. A graphical dermatome map is also captured via the iPad system to illustrate the distribution of the rash and evaluate whether it confirms to 1 or multiple dermatomes. These images are automatically incorporated into the study database and can be sent immediately to the trial's safety monitor and, as needed, to the Data Safety and Monitoring Board or an event adjudication committee.

DATA LINKAGES

The VERVE trial requires only two in-person study visits, greatly increasing efficiency, reducing cost, and decreasing both study site and participant burden. The longer-term effectiveness of the vaccine to prevent varicella zoster virus reactivation (ie, shingles), however, is also of high interest. Therefore, efficient collection of long-term outcome data on the incidence of shingles in the vaccinated versus unvaccinated patients is important. Moreover, it might be useful to obtain similar information for patients who were eligible for the trial but elected not to participate and on those who were never approached to participate. These two additional comparator groups can provide additional information regarding the generalizability of the trial's intervention to the population to which the intervention ultimately will be applied. Through data linkage, this information and other information from different sources (eg, administrative claims) can be integrated and a richer and more complete data set can be generated.

Sources of Linkable Data for Trial Outcome Ascertainment

A variety of data sources are available to assist in generation of RWE, and these can be potentially linked to one another. Examples of potential sources of data that can inform research (and clinical care) are shown in **Fig. 4**. Although each of these has both strengths and weakness as a data source, the strengths of one data source can potentially be used to fill in the gaps in the others and supplement the data collection efforts of the trial. For safety outcomes or clinical outcomes, for example, administrative claims data from commercial health plans or governmental sources (eg, the US Medicare program) can provide a highly efficient method for case ascertainment.

Certain types of events have been shown to be accurately ascertained in administrative claims data, based on algorithms validated against medical records as the gold standard. Examples of these outcomes and their validity as ascertained in high-quality validation studies are shown in **Table 1**. The potential benefit to this approach is that this linkage is passive, requiring no additional study visits and reducing participant and site burden and trial costs. If the positive predictive value of these events is high enough (eg, 85% or better), this approach for case ascertainment might be used by itself. In contrast, if it is not that high, then the linked claims data might be used for initial case finding and then additional review (via the EMR or other forms of medical record retrieval), with adjudication as needed, can be conducted. This approach to use health plan claims data to augment case ascertainment has been demonstrated successfully in linkages with traditional registries[25–27] and observational studies that satisfy FDA regulatory requirements.[28] This approach also can be used to support long-term safety and clinical outcome assessment in pragmatic trials. For example, a linkage with administrative health plan data was coupled to the Women's Health Initiative trial and was found able to yield essentially the same trial result as the much costlier and labor-intensive cardiovascular case ascertainment and clinical

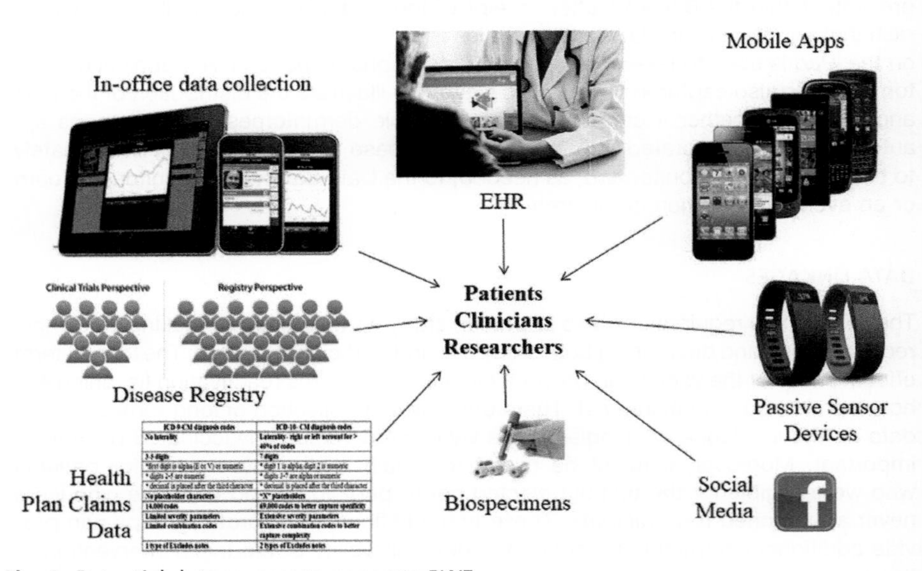

Fig. 4. Potential data sources to generate RWE.

Table 1
Clinical events and outcomes that can be ascertained with high validity[a] using administrative data[44]

Event Type	Selected Examples in Rheumatology
Myocardial infarction	Kim et al,[45] 2017; Xie et al,[46] 2018
Stroke	Kim et al,[45] 2017; Xie et al,[46] 2018
Cardiovascular death	Xie et al,[46] 2018
Herpes zoster	Curtis et al,[47] 2018; Cheetham et al,[48] 2015
Gastrointestinal bleeding	Le et al,[49] 2013
Interstitial lung disease	Le et al,[49] 2013; Curtis et al,[50] 2015
Gastrointestinal perforation	Xie et al,[51] 2016
Vertebral and nonvertebral fracture	Balasubramanian et al,[52] 2019
Malignancy	Setoguchi et al,[53] 2006
Medical procedures (eg, joint replacement)	George et al,[54] 2017
Costs	Curtis et al,[55] 2017
Death	Curtis et al,[55] 2017; England et al,[56] 2018

[a] Based on the existence of 1 or more high-quality validation studies comparing an administrative data-based algorithm to the gold standard of medical record review with adjudication.

Data from West SL, Storm BL, Poole C. Validity of pharmacoepidemiologic drug and diagnosis data. In: Strom BL, editor. Pharmacoepidemiology. 4th edition. West Sussex (England): Wiley; 2005. p. 743–55.

adjudication that was principally used for the Women's Health Initiative trial.[29,30] This capacity was also built into the VERVE trial to facilitate long-term case ascertainment for herpes zoster events (discussed later).

Data Linkage in the VaricEcella zosteR VaccinE Trial

In addition to facilitating obtaining informed consent from participants, the tablet-based system, described previously, that was implemented in the VERVE trial, also digitally captured identifiable information that could be used to link to health plan data (eg, Social Security number), such as Medicare, commercial claims data, or EMR data sources. Because the validity of case identification for herpes zoster reactivation is high (positive predictive value 85%–100%) in these data sources,[31–34] explicit in-person study visits to capture these events may not be required, reducing costs and minimizing participant burden. If administrative claims data are used for case ascertainment (eg, *International Classification of Diseases*, *Ninth Revision*/*International Classification of Diseases*, *Tenth Revision* code for herpes zoster plus proximate receipt of an antiviral medication commonly used to treatment varicella) yet additional clinical information is desired, information from medical record can be obtained.

To this end, the patient's signature collected digitally in VERVE also satisfied the requirements for HIPAA authorization and was used to populate a study-specific medical record release form. The purpose of the medical record release form was to enable centralized safety follow-up, including medical record retrieval, for serious adverse events and for shingles. Specifically, if a serious adverse event occurred after 6 weeks, the VERVE call center (run by FORWARD, the National Data Bank for Rheumatic Diseases) was responsible for obtaining the relevant information, including medical records from a provider or a hospital. If medical records were required, the electronically signed medical record release form, therefore, would already be available to the call center to facilitate retrieval.

In addition to the capacity to identify herpes zoster cases among trial participants using passive claims or EMR data sources, data linkage facilitates ascertainment of herpes zoster outcome events in nonparticipants. This includes both those who might have been approached at the trial site but who did not participate, as well those receiving care at sites not participating in the trial. This approach, using both data sources, helps to inform generalizability of the trial's outcomes to the broader patient population of individuals who might benefit from the intervention.

Technical Aspects to Data Linkage—The Role of Unique Identifiers and Other Probabilistic Approaches

Although VERVE collected trial participants' social security number to facilitate data linkage with national claims and EMR data, there are many circumstances where participants are unwilling to provide this information. Other sensitive identifiers (eg, health insurance number) also may provoke similar reluctance for sharing. For that reason, a variety of less sensitive and nonunique identifiers can be collected to facilitate data linkage. For example, the combination of name, gender, date of birth, health care provider (eg, US physician's national provider ID[35] or hospital identifier), and 1 or more event dates (eg, date of physician office visit, hospital admission, or device implantation) has been shown to facilitate data linkage between claims data and a research registry with high accuracy.[36] Linkage can be done with either deterministic (ie, rule-based) or probabilistic methods. Patient names likely need to be normalized to remove spaces and truncate them (eg, using the first 2 digits), because name misspellings, colloquialisms (eg, Rob rather than Robert), suffixes (eg, Jr. and Sr.), and spacing variability (eg, van der Heidje vs vanDerHeidje) reduce the sensitivity of matching based on full name. In one study,[37] a composite identifier based on truncated name and date of birth was shown to have good performance characteristics (sensitivity 97%; specificity approaching 100%) and outperformed linkage based on social security number. It also had much better sensitivity than linkage on full name and date of birth (sensitivity 87%). Evaluating this concept in the context of a university health system providing care to approximately 3 million patients, and adding in information regarding physician National Provider Identifier as a potential identifier, the specificity of a composite identifier consisting of the first 2 digits of patient first and last names, middle initial, date of birth, gender, and National Provider Identifier yielded specificity of greater than 99.8%.[38]

Although health systems and medical providers are generally willing to share identifiable information if patients have explicitly consented to such disclosure, there are other research-related use cases (including pragmatic trials) where consent may not be feasible to obtain or was considered only after the fact and is not possible to obtain post hoc. Therefore, health systems and other covered entities would be appropriately reluctant or unable to share any personal identifying information (PII). A third-party honest broker sometimes can be engaged to serve in role of a trusted intermediary whose sole function is to identify and link patients between 2 or more data systems based on PII but who are given no other health information (ie, personal health information [PHI]).[39] As an alternative, cryptographic hashing approaches can be used to link patients. A hash function takes an input string (eg, a set of patient identifiers) that applies a mathematical algorithm to create a string of a fixed size. This is typically 1-way, which means that it cannot be used to reconstruct the original input string. The properties of an optimal hash function include the expectation that it is deterministic (ie, the same inputs always result in the same hash string output), it is unique (different input strings should yield unique hash output strings), and the hashed output is uncorrelated with its input string, so that small changes in the input string generally result in

Table 2
Examples of hashing, salting, and encryption to facilitate data linkage, as used in a rheumatology-specific, iPad-based app (READY) to collect patient-reported outcome data in rheumatology clinics

Process	First Name	Last Name	Gender	Date of Birth	Hashed Identifier (1-Way Hash)	Visit Date	Encrypted	Observation Period	Day Offset[a]	Patient-reported Outcome Score (eg, Fatigue)
Data input into READY app	Iron	Man	M	1/1/1960	—	3/1/2018	—	—	—	55
Stored by READY within AWS	—	—	—	—	5e6376106b14700d775 cfef3a62cad21ee3e6a baf579e811778813 ec09fffc6c	vEr2qZ9Ar1zPIX w731WGnBo0f LPPgYyULeo8o GZDt5s=	Yes	—	—	55
Available within AWS aftaer decryption and prior to deidentification	—	—	—	—	5e6376106b14700d775cf ef3a62cad21ee3e6aba f579e811778813ec09fffc6c	3/1/2018	No	—	—	55
Deidentified data set	—	—	—	—	5e6376106b14700d77 5cfef3a62cad21ee3e 6abaf579e81177881 3ec09fffc6c	—	—	2018Q1[a]	0	55

Note: no other personal identifiers are stored in AWS. The above example is exhaustive with respect to identifiers that relate to individual patients.

Abbreviations: —, Signifies null/blank; AWS, Amazon web services. READY, RhEumAtic Disease activitY.

[a] The visit date is converted into an offset based on the number of days since the date of each individual's first observation in the database, which is arbitrarily set as day 0.

Data from Mathur P, Embi PJ, Cutis JR. Pages. Accessed at iTunes at. Available at: https://itunes.apple.com/us/app/rheumatic-disease-activity/id657411562?mt=8. Accessed January 24, 2019.

major changes in the output string. A vector of patient identifiers that will be used to create the hash must first be decided on. This can then be salted by concatenating an additional customized phrase to the input string to foil a dictionary attack. If dates must be stored (which are allowed under the rules applicable to a limited data set), they can be encrypted but then transformed to a fully deidentified data set by setting the first observation to be an arbitrary day 0 and representing every subsequent date as the number of days offset from day 0. An example from actual implementation of a tablet-based (iPad) system used to collect patient-reported outcome data in a rheumatology clinic setting[40,41] is shown in **Table 2**. The hashed string is generated by both parties and can be exchanged (because it can no longer be linked back to an individual) and then linked via deterministic methods to match patients uniquely between the data sources.

As a final concept and a limitation to the cryptographic hashing approach, the process is essentially a black box and lacks verifiability of the accuracy of the approach, with opaqueness around both its sensitivity and specificity for any given linkage use case. For that reason, additional privacy-conserving methods to enable and verify high-quality linkage, enable minimal PII and PHI disclosure, and monitor for drifts in data linkage have been developed.[42] This approach can take various forms, but, for example, it might highlight data only where differences in the PII between potentially linked patients exist but not disclose the actual differences in the PII. This enables partial disclosure and only for data elements that are necessary. The process also can support manual review for key subgroups of potentially linked matched pairs where greater uncertainty exists, increasing confidence both in the process and in its result.

SUMMARY

A variety of tools and approaches are needed to support efficient generation of high-quality, RWE to support research and promote high-quality clinical care. Pragmatic trials; digital data capture, including electronic consent; and linkages between data sources can facilitate these efficiencies to support the next generation of research both for rheumatology and more broadly. In addition, through platforms like SMART IRB, and with updated NIH guidance, and recent changes to the Common Rule, the IRB process is becoming more efficient, creating cost and time savings for those interested in efficient RWE generation. Innovations such as these in clinical trial design have the potential to allow larger, more generalizable, and more cost-effective studies that ultimate better guide real-world care.

REFERENCES

1. Sherman RE, Anderson SA, Dal Pan GJ, et al. Real-world evidence - what is it and what can it tell us? N Engl J Med 2016;375(23):2293–7.
2. Greenberg JD, Kishimoto M, Strand V, et al. Tumor necrosis factor antagonist responsiveness in a United States rheumatoid arthritis cohort. Am J Med 2008; 121(6):532–8.
3. Vashisht P, Sayles H, Cannella AC, et al. Generalizability of patients with rheumatoid arthritis in biologic agent clinical trials. Arthritis Care Res (Hoboken) 2016; 68(10):1478–88.
4. Harrold LR, Reed GW, John A, et al. Cluster-randomized trial of a behavioral intervention to incorporate a treat-to-target approach to care of us patients with rheumatoid arthritis. Arthritis Care Res (Hoboken) 2018;70(3):379–87.
5. 21st Century Cures Act, Pub. L. 114 - 255, 130 Stat. 1033 (2016).

6. Zwarenstein M, Treweek S, Gagnier JJ, et al. Improving the reporting of pragmatic trials: an extension of the CONSORT statement. BMJ 2008;337:a2390.
7. Loudon K, Treweek S, Sullivan F, et al. The PRECIS-2 tool: designing trials that are fit for purpose. BMJ 2015;350:h2147.
8. Reynolds RF, Lem JA, Gatto NM, et al. Is the large simple trial design used for comparative, post-approval safety research? A review of a clinical trials registry and the published literature. Drug Saf 2011;34(10):799–820.
9. Strom BL, Faich GA, Reynolds RF, et al. The Ziprasidone Observational Study of Cardiac Outcomes (ZODIAC): design and baseline subject characteristics. J Clin Psychiatry 2008;69(1):114–21.
10. ALLHAT Officers and Coordinators for the ALLHAT Collaborative Research Group, The Antihypertensive and Lipid-Lowering Treatment to Prevent Heart Attack Trial. Major outcomes in moderately hypercholesterolemic, hypertensive patients randomized to pravastatin vs usual care: The Antihypertensive and Lipid-Lowering Treatment to Prevent Heart Attack Trial (ALLHAT-LLT). JAMA 2002;288(23):2998–3007.
11. Mikuls TR, Cheetham TC, Levy GD, et al. Adherence and outcomes with urate-lowering therapy: a site-randomized trial. Am J Med 2018. [Epub ahead of print].
12. ClinicalTrials.gov. 2015. Available at: Pages https://clinicaltrials.gov/ct2/show/NCT02538341. Accessed January 23, 2019.
13. i2b2.org 2019;Pages. Accessed at A National Center for Biomedical Computing Available at: https://www.i2b2.org/resrcs/. Accessed January 24, 2019.
14. TransmartFoundation.org. 2019. Available at: Pages https://transmartfoundation.org/. Accessed January 24, 2019.
15. U.S. Department of Health and Human Services, National Institutes of Health. (2017). Single IRB Policy for Multi-site Research (NIH Publication No. NOT-OD-16-094). Retrieved from https://grants.nih.gov/grants/policy/faq_single_IRB_policy_research.htm.
16. Messner DA, Moloney R, Warriner AH, et al. Understanding practice-based research participation: The differing motivations of engaged vs. non-engaged clinicians in pragmatic clinical trials. Contemp Clin Trials Commun 2016;4:136–40.
17. Williams CM, Maher CG, Hancock MJ, et al. Recruitment rate for a clinical trial was associated with particular operational procedures and clinician characteristics. J Clin Epidemiol 2014;67(2):169–75.
18. Eapen ZJ, Lauer MS, Temple RJ. The imperative of overcoming barriers to the conduct of large, simple trials. JAMA 2014;311(14):1397–8.
19. Warner ET, Glasgow RE, Emmons KM, et al. Recruitment and retention of participants in a pragmatic randomized intervention trial at three community health clinics: results and lessons learned. BMC Public Health 2013;13:192.
20. Wright NC, Foster PJ, Mudano AS, et al. Assessing the feasibility of the Effectiveness of Discontinuing Bisphosphonates trial: a pilot study. Osteoporos Int 2017;28(8):2495–503.
21. California State Assembly. Protection of human subjects in medical experimentation act.1978 Session of the Legislature. Statutes of California. State of California. Ch. 360 p. 24170 - 24179.5.
22. Justice SoCDo 2019;Pages. Accessed at Office of the Attorney General Available at: https://oag.ca.gov/research/consent. Accessed January 23, 2019.
23. Warriner AH, Foster PJ, Mudano A, et al. A pragmatic randomized trial comparing tablet computer informed consent to traditional paper-based methods for an osteoporosis study. Contemp Clin Trials Commun 2016;3:32–8.

24. US Department of Health & Human Services. Use of electronic informed consent: questions and answers (HSS Publication 45 CFR part 46). 2016. Available at: https://www.hhs.gov/ohrp/regulations-and-policy/guidance/use-electronic-informed-consent-questions-and-answers/index.html.
25. Curtis JR, Baddley JW, Yang S, et al. Derivation and preliminary validation of an administrative claims-based algorithm for the effectiveness of medications for rheumatoid arthritis. Arthritis Res Ther 2011;13(5):R155.
26. Kumamaru H, Judd SE, Curtis JR, et al. Validity of claims-based stroke algorithms in contemporary Medicare data: reasons for geographic and racial differences in stroke (REGARDS) study linked with medicare claims. Circ Cardiovasc Qual Outcomes 2014;7(4):611–9.
27. Schousboe JT, Paudel ML, Taylor BC, et al. Magnitude and consequences of misclassification of incident hip fractures in large cohort studies: the Study of Osteoporotic Fractures and Medicare claims data. Osteoporos Int 2013;24(3): 801–10.
28. Xue F, Ma H, Stehman-Breen C, et al. Design and methods of a postmarketing pharmacoepidemiology study assessing long-term safety of Prolia(R) (denosumab) for the treatment of postmenopausal osteoporosis. Pharmacoepidemiol Drug Saf 2013;22(10):1107–14.
29. Lakshminarayan K, Larson JC, Virnig B, et al. Comparison of Medicare claims versus physician adjudication for identifying stroke outcomes in the women's health initiative. Stroke 2014;45(3):815–21.
30. Hlatky MA, Ray RM, Burwen DR, et al. Use of Medicare data to identify coronary heart disease outcomes in the Women's Health Initiative. Circ Cardiovasc Qual Outcomes 2014;7(1):157–62.
31. Yawn BP, Gilden D. The global epidemiology of herpes zoster. Neurology 2013; 81(10):928–30.
32. Baxter R, Bartlett J, Fireman B, et al. Long-term effectiveness of the live zoster vaccine in preventing shingles: a cohort study. Am J Epidemiol 2018;187(1): 161–9.
33. Galil K, Choo PW, Donahue JG, et al. The sequelae of herpes zoster. Arch Intern Med 1997;157(11):1209–13.
34. Donahue JG, Choo PW, Manson JE, et al. The incidence of herpes zoster. Arch Intern Med 1995;155(15):1605–9.
35. Available at: CMS.gov; Pages https://www.cms.gov/Regulations-and-Guidance/Administrative-Simplification/NationalProvIdentStand/DataDissemination.html. Accessed January 23, 2019.
36. Curtis JR, Chen L, Bharat A, et al. Linkage of a de-identified United States rheumatoid arthritis registry with administrative data to facilitate comparative effectiveness research. Arthritis Care Res (Hoboken) 2014;66(12):1790–8.
37. Weber SC, Lowe H, Das A, et al. A simple heuristic for blindfolded record linkage. J Am Med Inform Assoc 2012;19(e1):e157–61.
38. Mathur P, SL, Bharat A. High Level Architecture and Evaluation of Patient Linkages for READY - An Electronic Measurement Tool for Rheumatoid Arthritis. AMIA Annual Symposium Proceedings San Francisco, CA; November 13-18, 2015.
39. Choi HJ, Lee MJ, Choi CM, et al. Establishing the role of honest broker: bridging the gap between protecting personal health data and clinical research efficiency. Peer J 2015;3:e1506.

40. Yen PY, Lara B, Lopetegui M, et al. Usability and workflow evaluation of "RhEumAtic Disease activitY" (READY). A mobile application for rheumatology patients and providers. Appl Clin Inform 2016;7(4):1007–24.
41. Mathur P, Embi PJ, Cutis JR. Pages. Accessed at iTunes at Available at: https://itunes.apple.com/us/app/rheumatic-disease-activity/id657411562?mt=8. Accessed January 24, 2019.
42. Kum HC, Krishnamurthy A, Machanavajjhala A, et al. Privacy preserving interactive record linkage (PPIRL). J Am Med Inform Assoc 2014;21(2):212–20.
43. Black DM, Schwartz AV, Ensrud KE, et al. Effects of continuing or stopping alendronate after 5 years of treatment: the Fracture Intervention Trial Long-term Extension (FLEX): a randomized trial. JAMA 2006;296(24):2927–38.
44. West SL, Storm BL, Poole C. Validity of Pharmacoepidemiologic Drug and Diagnosis Data. In: Strom BL, editor. Pharmacoepidemiology. 4th edition. West Sussex, England: Wiley; 2005. p. 743–55.
45. Kim SC, Solomon DH, Rogers JR, et al. Cardiovascular Safety of tocilizumab versus tumor necrosis factor inhibitors in patients with rheumatoid arthritis: a multi-database cohort study. Arthritis Rheumatol 2017;69(6):1154–64.
46. Xie F, Yun H, Levitan EB, et al. Tocilizumab and the risk for cardiovascular disease: a direct comparison among biologic disease-modifying antirheumatic drugs for rheumatoid arthritis patients. Arthritis Care Res (Hoboken) 2018. [Epub ahead of print].
47. Curtis JR, Xie F, Yang S, et al. Herpes zoster in tofacitinib: risk is further increased with glucocorticoids but not methotrexate. Arthritis Care Res (Hoboken) 2018. [Epub ahead of print].
48. Cheetham TC, Marcy SM, Tseng HF, et al. Risk of herpes zoster and disseminated varicella zoster in patients taking immunosuppressant drugs at the time of zoster vaccination. Mayo Clin Proc 2015;90(7):865–73.
49. Le HV, Poole C, Brookhart MA, et al. Effects of aggregation of drug and diagnostic codes on the performance of the high-dimensional propensity score algorithm: an empirical example. BMC Med Res Methodol 2013;13:142.
50. Curtis JR, Sarsour K, Napalkov P, et al. Incidence and complications of interstitial lung disease in users of tocilizumab, rituximab, abatacept and anti-tumor necrosis factor alpha agents, a retrospective cohort study. Arthritis Res Ther 2015;17:319.
51. Xie F, Yun H, Bernatsky S, et al. Brief report: risk of gastrointestinal perforation among rheumatoid arthritis patients receiving tofacitinib, tocilizumab, or other biologic treatments. Arthritis Rheumatol 2016;68(11):2612–7.
52. Balasubramanian A, Zhang J, Chen L, et al. Risk of subsequent fracture after prior fracture among older women. Osteoporos Int 2019;30(1):79–92.
53. Setoguchi S, Solomon DH, Weinblatt ME, et al. Tumor necrosis factor alpha antagonist use and cancer in patients with rheumatoid arthritis. Arthritis Rheum 2006;54(9):2757–64.
54. George MD, Baker JF, Hsu JY, et al. Perioperative timing of infliximab and the risk of serious infection after elective hip and knee arthroplasty. Arthritis Care Res (Hoboken) 2017;69(12):1845–54.
55. Curtis JR, Chen L, Greenberg JD, et al. The clinical status and economic savings associated with remission among patients with rheumatoid arthritis: leveraging linked registry and claims data for synergistic insights. Pharmacoepidemiol Drug Saf 2017;26(3):310–9.
56. England BR, Sayles H, Michaud K, et al. Chronic lung disease in U.S. Veterans with rheumatoid arthritis and the impact on survival. Clin Rheumatol 2018; 37(11):2907–15.

40. Yen PY, Lara B, Lopetegui M, et al. Usability and workflow evaluation of "RhEumAtic Disease activitY" (READY). A mobile application for rheumatology patients and providers. Appl Clin Inform 2016;7(4):1007–24.
41. Malton P, Emery P, Curtis JR. Pages. Accessed at iTunes. Available at: https://itunes.apple.com/us/app/rheumatic-disease-activity/id1094571928?mt=8. Accessed January 24, 2019.
42. Kum HC, Krishnamurthy A, Machanavajjhala A, et al. Privacy preserving interactive record linkage (PPIRL). J Am Med Inform Assoc 2014;21(2):212–20.
43. Black DM, Schwartz AV, Ensrud KE, et al. Effects of continuing or stopping alendronate after 5 years of treatment: the Fracture Intervention Trial Long-term Extension (FLEX): a randomized trial. JAMA 2006;296(24):2927–38.
44. West SL, Strom BL, Poole C. Validity of Pharmacoepidemiologic Drug and Diagnosis Data. In: Strom BL, editor. Pharmacoepidemiology. 4th edition. West Sussex, England: Wiley; 2005. p. 709–65.
45. Kim SC, Solomon DH, Rogers JR, et al. Cardiovascular Safety of tocilizumab versus tumor necrosis factor inhibitors in patients with rheumatoid arthritis: a multi-database cohort study. Arthritis Rheumatol 2017;69(6):1154–64.
46. Xie F, Yun H, Levitan EB, et al. Tocilizumab and the risk for cardiovascular disease: a direct comparison among biologic disease-modifying antirheumatic drugs for rheumatoid arthritis patients. Arthritis Care Res (Hoboken) 2019. [Epub ahead of print].
47. Curtis JR, Xie F, Yang S, et al. Herpes zoster in tofacitinib: risk is further increased with glucocorticoids but not methotrexate. Arthritis Care Res (Hoboken) 2019. [Epub ahead of print].
48. Cheetham TC, Marcy SM, Tseng HF, et al. Risk of herpes zoster and disseminated varicella zoster in patients taking immunosuppressant drugs at the time of zoster vaccination. Mayo Clin Proc 2015;90(7):865–73.
49. Le HV, Poole C, Brookhart MA, et al. Effects of aggregation of drug and diagnostic codes on the performance of the high-dimensional propensity score algorithm: an empirical example. BMC Med Res Methodol 2013;13:142.
50. Curtis JR, Sarsour K, Napalkov P, et al. Incidence and complications of interstitial lung disease in users of tocilizumab, rituximab, abatacept and anti-tumor necrosis factor alpha agents, a retrospective cohort study. Arthritis Res Ther 2015;17:319.
51. Xie F, Yun H, Bernatsky S, et al. Brief report: risk of gastrointestinal perforation among rheumatoid arthritis patients receiving tofacitinib, tocilizumab, or other biologic treatments. Arthritis Rheumatol 2016;68(11):2612–7.
52. Balasubramanian A, Zhang J, Chen L, et al. Risk of subsequent fracture after prior fracture among older women. Osteoporos Int 2019;30(1):79–92.
53. Setoguchi S, Solomon DH, Weinblatt ME, et al. Tumor necrosis factor alpha antagonist use and cancer in patients with rheumatoid arthritis. Arthritis Rheum 2006;54(9):2757–64.
54. George MD, Baker JF, Hsu JY, et al. Perioperative timing of infliximab and the risk of serious infection after elective hip and knee arthroplasty. Arthritis Care Res (Hoboken) 2017;69(12):1845–54.
55. Curtis JR, Chen L, Greenberg JD, et al. The clinical status and economic savings associated with remission among patients with rheumatoid arthritis: leveraging linked registry and claims data for synergistic insights. Pharmacoepidemiol Drug Saf 2017;26(3):310–9.
56. England BR, Sayles H, Michaud K, et al. Chronic lung disease in U.S. veterans with rheumatoid arthritis and the impact on survival. Clin Rheumatol 2018;37(11):2907–15.

Imaging in the Mobile Domain

Paul Bird, PhD, GradDipMRI, FRACP

KEYWORDS

- Mobile imaging applications • Battlefield MRI • SQUIDs • OsiriX

KEY POINTS

- Mobile imaging data encompasses programs that facilitate the ability for physicians to view images on a smart phone application, tablet, or desktop, and share those images with colleagues.
- Mobile MIM software and OsiriX software are 2 examples of imaging processing software. Both illustrate different aspects of imaging software.
- The advent of capacitive micromachine ultrasound transducers within the ultrasound transducer is an example of changing technology, potentially providing portable, cost-effective, and accessible ultrasound examinations.
- Ultra low field MRI, based on a battlefield MRI model that incorporates super conducting quantum interference devices, allows ultra low field MRI bypassing the limitations of high field MRI. This modality has the potential to allow MRI access in remote areas with transfer of images for central reading.
- Artificial intelligence will assist in image segmentation, diagnosis, detection of lesions, and the monitoring of therapy in conjunction with human endeavors.

INTRODUCTION

Mobile is usually used as an adjective—an object or entity that can move or be moved freely or easily. Considering imaging, the concept of mobility can be separated into 2 areas. The first is the transfer of images, for comparison, interpretation, or teaching. In a modern world, fast and accurate transfer of images is essential so that we have access to them when required. The second is the mobility of imaging devices—not necessarily simply smaller, portable imaging devices, but also tools that are more accessible, easier to use by persons without advanced training, and with wider application.

Disclosure: P. Bird has provided consultative services to Bioclinica, Boston Imaging Core Lab, and Synarc. The author has no financial relationship with the applications or imaging hardware presented in this article. The author has no conflict to declare in this regard.

University of New South Wales, Suite 4 Level 1, 19 Kensington Street, Kogarah, Sydney, New South Wales 2217, Australia
E-mail address: p.bird@unsw.edu.au

Rheum Dis Clin N Am 45 (2019) 291–302
https://doi.org/10.1016/j.rdc.2019.01.002

The first part of this article examines some aspects of imaging software, with a focus on the currently available tools for images transfer, display, and interpretation. The discussion includes programs amenable to smartphone display as well as those suited to desktop performance. These include MIM software (MIM Software, Cleveland, OH), OsiriX (Pixmeo SARL, Bernex, Switzerland), Resolution MD (Calgary Scientific Inc, Calgary, Canada), iClarity (iClarity, Bellevue, WA), and eFilm (IBM Watson Health, Cambridge, MA). The second portion focuses on imaging devices, with the discussion centered around the potential of portable and accessible ultrasound examination, ultra low field MRI, and artificial intelligence (AI) in radiology.

PART 1

The Rise of Health Care Applications

Patients and physicians are increasingly aware of smart phone technology and applications as facilitators to assist health decisions and to assist health care delivery.[1] Data from US mHealth apps market shows an increasing trend in the general community to use of applications to facilitate medication adherence, nutrition choices, and exercise regimens.

Among US physicians, data suggest that smartphone apps are increasingly used to access drug information, communicate with nursing staff, access medical research, and access evidence-based clinical reference tools at the point of care.[2,3] These point-of-care resources are a growing adjunct to delivery of health care, and imaging fit well within this paradigm.

Rheumatologists are increasingly skilled in image interpretation, and images are often used to facilitate treatment decisions such as escalation of therapy. It follows that the ability to view an image at the point of care as a part of the decision-making process forms an important part of health care delivery for the modern physician.

Mobile Imaging Applications

Mobile imaging applications, by definition, allow image display on smartphones, a desktop, or a tablet at the point of care. Beyond the point of care, the mobile imaging application allows the presentation of images for review, easy image sharing for opinion, and rapid access to results away from the office environment.

Mobile imaging applications can be divided into 2 broad types. Applications of general usefulness that display imaging, have limited interpretation potential and may or may not be approved by the US Food and Drug Administration (FDA). Examples include Mobile MIM, iClarity, and Resolution 3D. These applications are suited to the general user, who may wish to view images but does not wish to undertake segmentation, sophisticated analysis, or interpretation. They are usually free or involve minimal user cost.

More advanced imaging programs are FDA approved, allow display of imaging as well as detailed analysis, segmentation, overlays, 3-dimensional (3D) rendering, and multifunction analysis. They are generally costly to purchase, have a yearly license fee, and have a lite version that is limited in functionality and low cost. Examples include OsiriX (**Fig. 1**) and eFilm.

There are a number of other specialized mobile radiology applications suited to radiologists, but less suited to physicians. Examples include Radiopedia, CME Epocrates, Doximity, Radiology 2.0, and A Night in The ER. All of these applications offer a higher level of information, sample cases, and functionality suited to the radiology trainee or radiologist, but are not included in the scope of this review.

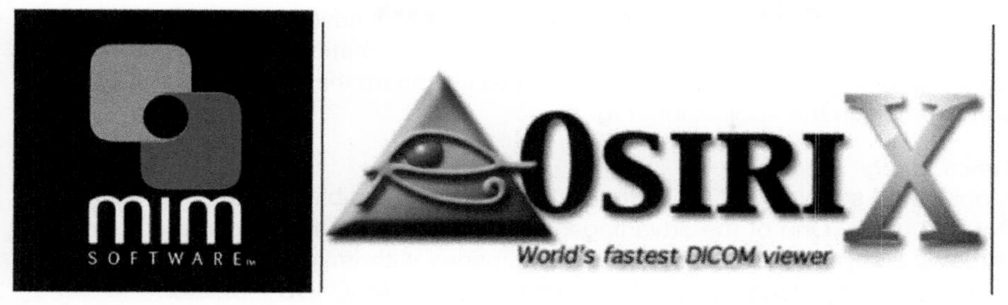

Fig. 1. Mobile imaging software applications—OsiriX and Mobile MIM. (*Courtesy of* Pixmeo.)

DIGITAL IMAGING AND COMMUNICATION IN MEDICINE

Digital imaging and communication in medicine (DICOM) is a worldwide standard for allowing the storing and transmitting information of medical images. The format provides a nonproprietary data interchange protocol and file structure for biomedical images and image related information, such as patient details.[4,5] The DICOM protocol is compatible with transmission control protocol and Internet protocol, meaning that DICOM application entities can be communicated over the Internet. DICOM originated initially in 1983 when the American College of Radiology and the National Electrical Manufacturers Association formed a Coalition and Standards Committee to standardize the needs of radiologists, radiographers, physicists, and equipment vendors with the first standard point-to-point image communication released in 1985.[6] Subsequently, after several iterations, the name was changed to DICOM in 1993 and over subsequent years DICOM has added formats for ultrasound examinations, x-ray angiography, CD, and MRI, as well as multiple other imaging modalities.

DICOM groups information into datasets that contain the patient's identifying information within the file so the image can never be separated by error. The benefit of DICOM is that it allows physicians and radiologists better access to images and reports when DICOM standards are in place and, as a result, DICOM forms the foundation for much of the imaging that we use currently.[5]

Importantly, mobile imaging applications using DICOM are widely available and the transfer of images using applications such as ultrasound examinations and MRI facilitates transfer of images over long distances using the DICOM format, meaning that imaging can be performed in remote locations and transferred for review.

MOBILE IMAGING APPLICATIONS USING DIGITAL IMAGING AND COMMUNICATION IN MEDICINE

Rather than list a large number of mobile imaging applications, this review focuses on 2 applications that best represent the general user interface and the more advanced user interface.

General User Interface: Mobile MIM

Description

Mobile MIM was one of the initial application in Apple's App Store in 2008. Later, the application was temporarily removed from the store while the program underwent regulatory assessment. After this assessment had been undertaken, the FDA granted the mobile radiology application a 510(k) clearance in 2011.[7] This clearance means that the Mobile MIM software is FDA approved for viewing images and making medical diagnoses based on CT scans, MRIs, ultrasound examinations, and PET images. The application is not intended to replace a standard work station, but to enable clinicians to view and display images on mobile devices and share these images easily using the software within the application (**Fig. 2**).

Functionality

Mobile MIM software is MAC, iPhone, and iPad compatible only and not suitable for Android users. One of the advantages of the software is that it is free and provides wireless and portable access to medical images with image data being transferred to the device by cloud servers. It is compatible with MAC IOS 7 or later.

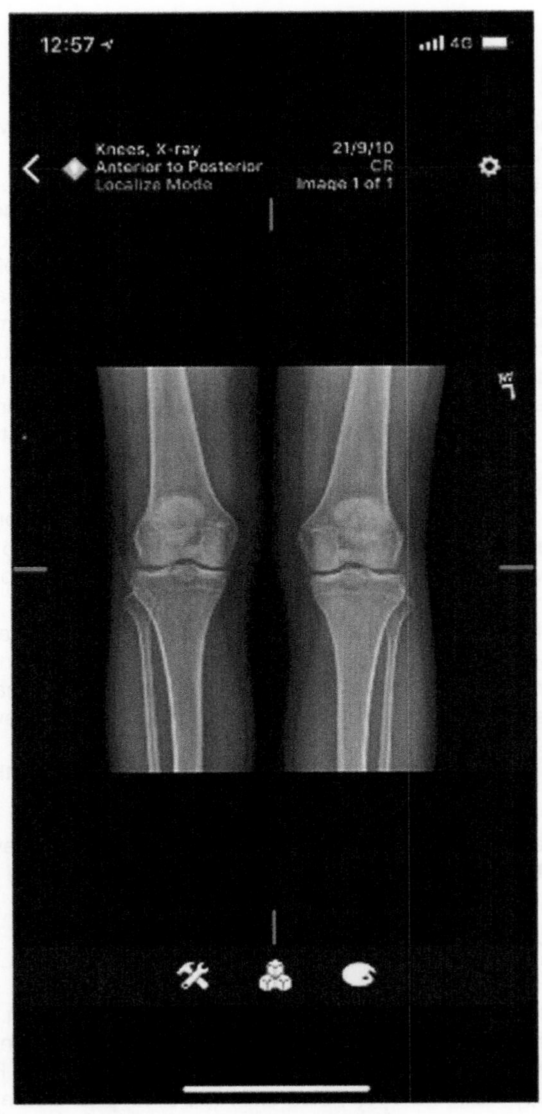

Fig. 2. Mobile MIM. Sample radiograph display smartphone.

Key functions

- Safety guide for clinicians to be completed before use ensures understanding of software.
- Images can be used and, by using Breeze Image Sharing, images can be shared.
- Within the software users can use several different tools to allow the fusion of software with 3D display with images being able to be stored in the cloud.

Use in clinical practice

Mobile MIM provides a free, utility-based software program that includes an interactive setup and mitigates the risk of poor image display owing to improper screen luminescence or lighting conditions. In the current form, the application provides some viewing capabilities, but does not replace a desktop application for image segmentation, diagnosis, and monitoring.

Advanced user interface

OsiriX

Description OsiriX software (**Fig. 3**) is a MAC-based program that provides 2 options for users. OsiriX MD is the complete edition of OsiriX, allowing not only the display and sharing of images on an iPhone, iPad, and desktop, but also allows advanced postprocessing techniques in 2 and 3 dimensions. Importantly, it can display any medical images (DICOM files) from a CD, DVD, USB stick, and website, and it has also been certified and validated for clinical use in medicine by the FDA.[8]

OsiriX Light is a free version that has less functionality than OsiriX MD. Osirix Lite is a good introduction to the program basics, but does not allow complete functionality, limited postprocessing software, and a limited number of images displayed; it is not FDA approved. OsirixMD is FDA cleared/CE labeled version for primary diagnostic imaging.

Functionality OsiriX was developed by the Pixmeo company based in Geneva and is an image processing software dedicated to DICOM images (.dcm/.DCM extension) produced by imaging equipment (MRI, computed tomography [CT], PET, PET-CT,

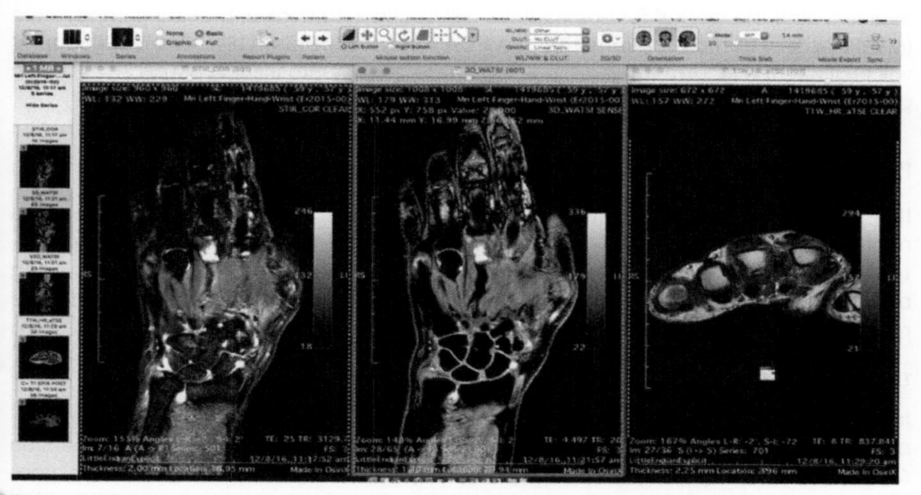

Fig. 3. OsiriX. Representative image from desktop demonstrating multitask tool bar, image display, and segmentation tools. (*Courtesy of* Pixmeo.)

single photon emission CT-CT, and ultrasound). The program can handle images transferred by DICOM communication protocol from any PACS or imaging modality.[9] OsiriX has been specifically designed for use as a DICOM PACS workstation for imaging and an image processing software for medical research, navigation, and visualization of multimodality and multidimensional images.[9]

Key functions OsiriX MD provides full functionality image processing for diagnostic purposes and advanced image processing techniques.

- A 2-dimensional viewer, 3D viewer, 4-dimensional viewer (3D series with temporal dimension; eg, cardiac CT), and 5-dimensional VIEWER (3D series with temporal and functional dimensions; eg, cardiac PET-CT).[10]
- Multiplanar reconstruction, surface rendering, volume rendering, and maximum intensity projection. All these modes support 4-dimensional data and are able to produce image fusion between 2 different series (PET-CT and single photon emission CT-CT display support).
- Thick slab for multislice CT and MRI (mean, maximum intensity projection, and volume rendering).
- Regions of interest: polygons, circles, pencil, rectangles, point—multiple tools to allow image segmentation with 3D volume calculation.
- Hanging protocols: This is the series of actions performed to arrange images for optimal viewing. The term originally referred to the arrangement of physical films on a light box or hanging of films on a film alternator. Now the term also includes the concept of displaying softcopy images on a PACS workstation. This concept is very important for readers in clinical trials.

Use in clinical practice In rheumatology, Osirix is used primarily to display, share, and segment images after processing. For imaging researchers, it is an important tool to facilitate image interpretation and segmentation, and has been used in several clinical trials and in specialized clinical practice scenarios.[11–13]

Summary

Two imaging applications have been reviewed in this article, but there are multiple available and the market for applications will continue to evolve, providing consumers (physicians) with more options that are FDA approved. Potentially, this development will facilitate the incorporation of imaging interpretation into clinical practice, assisting point-of-care treatment decisions.

PART 2: MOBILE IMAGING DEVICES

It is important to note that the technologies outlined in this part of review are not a replacement for current, well-established ultrasound and MRI protocols in rheumatology. The examples presented represent changes in the approach to these imaging methods, with the potential to augment current protocols in the future if proven to be reliable and valid.

Ultrasound Examination

In rheumatology, ultrasound examination has provided insights into subclinical pathology and has become an adjunct to clinical decision making with consensus papers on standardized procedures readily available.[10] Synovitis, bone erosions, and tenosynovitis are that can be assessed using ultrasound examination and ultrasound-guided joint injections form an increasing part of clinical practice for rheumatologists.[14]

Although well-recognized as a reliable and valid outcome measure in rheumatology clinical trials, ultrasound examination has several mobility disadvantages. These include the high cost of ultrasound machines, the lack of portable devices, and the need for advanced training to ensure that users are undertaking image acquisition correctly.[15] True mobile ultrasound imaging would encompass portable inexpensive devices that require limited training, interface with existing devices, and use AI to assist image acquisition for users with limited training.

Mobile ultrasound examination: technology innovations

Capacitive micromachine ultrasound transducers Capacitive micromachine ultrasound transducer (CMUT)-based ultrasound has emerged as a potential market disruptor in the ultrasound field, satisfying many of the requirements for true mobile imaging. This inexpensive, handheld ultrasound tool has FDA clearance[16] for 13 clinical applications, including cardiac scans, fetal and obstetric examinations, and musculoskeletal imaging (trade name Butterfly Ultrasound [Butterfly iQ, Guilford, CT]). The prospective advantage of the CMUT ultrasound system is that, rather than using a dedicated piece of hardware for image acquisition and display, the device interfaces with the users iPhone and the comparative cost is inexpensive. The baseline cost for a CMUT ultrasound (brand name Butterfly) is approximately USD $2000, compared with USD $50,000 for a standard piezoelectric crystal based ultrasound device.

The key to the portability and price decrease is the CMUT technology used for the transducer. Piezoelectric crystals are used in standard ultrasound transducer probes and convert electrical energy into vibrations in the form of ultrasonic energy, with a typical system having a display screen on a cart with several different probes for imaging at different depths and anatomic sites.[17] Smaller and more inexpensive devices have been developed (eg, GE Vscan products), but these devices have not significantly decrease the price to allow widespread access and, as the size decreases, the quality of the image decreases.

The CMUT (**Fig. 4**) challenges the piezoelectric model with a micro transducer that registers ultrasonic waves by moving the transducer membrane (akin to a drum) with the waves converted to an electrical signal, later converted to an image. Thousands of the micro machine transducers are included in a probe, which provides a very large

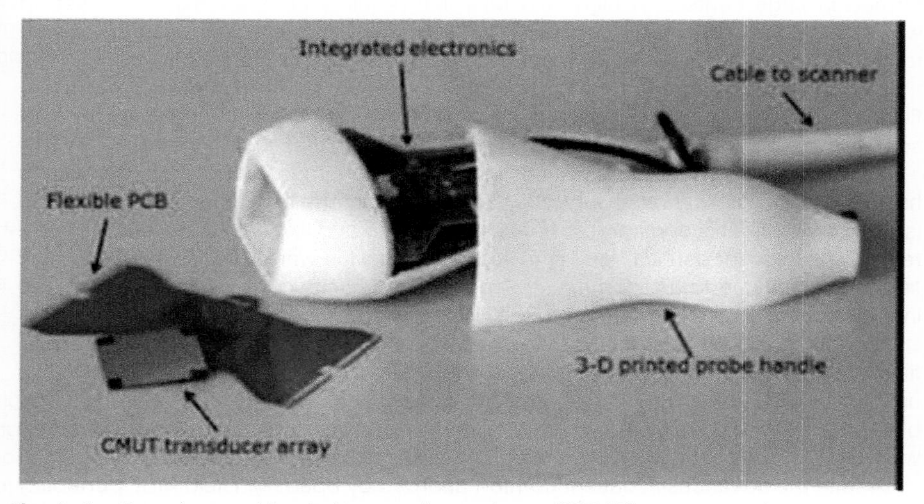

Fig. 4. Captive micromachined ultrasound transducers (CMUTs).

dynamic range, meaning that only 1 probe is required for all applications.[18] In addition, a typical piezoelectric probe is connected to electrical controls and displays by complicated wiring. The micro machine transducers are attached directly to a semi-conductive layer that contains all of the necessary amplifiers in a single process with simplified wiring.[19] This means that the CMUT ultrasound could potentially be a market disruptor for a number of reasons. The low cost improves accessibility, the portable nature of the device means it can be used in all environments, and there is a potential for less training being required to obtain high-quality images.

However, caution must be exercised. There is no evidence to date that CMUT technology can replace existing ultrasound methodology in rheumatology clinical practice or in trials. The rigorous assessment of such devices needs to be undertaken and, as the technology advances, rheumatologists and patients will require meticulously gathered evidence that modes such as power Doppler can be reproduced reliably in CMUT-based ultrasound models, and that the images thereafter produced do not compromise on quality. The feasibility, reliability, and validity all need to be assessed before the technology is embraced. But as a technological advance, CMUT technology represents a modification worthy of attention, and an area of advance that displays the future concept of true mobile imaging.

MRI: Ultra low field imaging

Standard MRI uses a powerful uniform external magnetic field used to align usually randomly orientated protons. The alignment is disrupted by external radiofrequency energy and the decay of signal or the relaxation time, used to produce an image by complex mathematical techniques. The most common MRI sequences used in rheumatology clinical trials are T1- and T2-weighted scans, with the T2-weighted sequence fat-suppressed using short T1 inversion recovery technique most commonly used.

MRI has shown usefulness in rheumatology for the early detection of erosions and joint space narrowing, and also has been used in large clinical trials for monitoring of the response to therapy, particularly with respect to synovitis, tenosynovitis, and osteitis.[20] Scoring systems exist for rheumatoid arthritis,[21] psoriatic arthritis,[22] and osteoarthritis.

Despite the advantages of MRI, the chief disadvantages are the high cost and the high-end technical aspects that require that the technique can usually only be performed in large centers. A high field MRI unit requires complex expensive set-up with shielding for the fringe magnetic field, as well as a highly skilled and trained staff to acquire images. This criterion limits the generalizability of the technique.

Low field MRI emerged in the early 2000s as an alternative to high field MRI. Low field extremity MRI provided advantages of comfort with a low fringe field and minimal set-up, meaning that the technique can be used in an office environment.

The OMERACT MRI group has investigated the advantages of low field MRI versus high field MRI. Publications have recorded that the interreliability for erosion scoring (static and change) is comparable between high field and low field units, but the inter-reader reliability for osteitis, tenosynovitis, and synovitis were less reliable.[23] As high field units continue to develop newer sequences the units continue to move forward in terms of image quality, leading to the development of open high field MRI.

Open high field MRI combines the benefit of safety with high field imaging. Vertical field open MRI provides excellent signal-to-noise ratio efficiency with greater signal uniformity. Additive arrangement gradient echo collects multiple echoes and combines them in the 1 acquisition, meaning that the common problems associated with short T1 inversion recovery images on low field can be circumvented.

Despite the advances in patient comfort afforded by open high field MRI, portability remains the major barrier to its widespread application. The search for alternate MRI techniques that would provide easy access in all situations led to the development of ultra low field MRI.

Battlefield MRI developed out of necessity in response to an increase in traumatic brain injury among service personnel during armed conflict in the early part of this century[24] High field magnets are not portable and, additionally, the risk of shrapnel in war zones limited the application of MRI in combatants suffering traumatic brain injury. The battlefield MRI was developed using super conducting quantum interference devices (SQUIDs), facilitating the detection of signal in ultra low magnetic fields.[25]

Super conducting quantum interference devices and ultra low magnetic field MRI

MRI at ultra low frequency has several advantages over conventional high field MRI. There is no contraindication in the presence of metal objects, as well as the possibility of achieving unique tissue contrasts and inflammation situations where a high magnetic field is simply impractical, such as war zones and in remote regions. The technology uses a magnetic field from 10 to 100 mT followed by a read-out at ultra low magnetic field using an ultrasensitive SQUID. The core of the ultra low field system is an SQUID sensor consisting of an SQUID coupled to a super conducting gradiometer.[26]

The magnetic field is applied to the lowest loop of the gradiometer, inducing a super current and, therefore, flux in the SQUID loop (**Fig. 5**). The flux transformer increases the sensitivity to nearby magnetic sources, providing a high level of rejection to distant magnetic sources, such as nearby radiation from cars or laboratory equipment. The gradiometer and SQUID are immersed in liquid helium to suppress the earth's field and external noise of the 3 layered shielding chamber.[27]

The major potential of the technique is the ability to used MRI in regions where the technology would simply not be available. As such, it embodies the theme of truly mobile imaging and is an area to watch with interest.

Ultra low field MRI is an emerging technology and, once again, it must be emphasized that the technology is not suggested as a replacement for standard MRI techniques and protocols. However, in changing the paradigm for image acquisition, ultra low field MRI represents an innovation born from necessity, and one that could potentially change the way that we acquire MR images in the future.

Artificial Intelligence in Radiology

AI in radiology has 2 major aspects: Machine learning algorithms based on predefined features and deep learning algorithms.

Machine learning algorithms based on predefined features

Traditional AI methods rely on predefined feature algorithms with parameters based on expert knowledge and epidemiologic information. Features within this category include the ability to identify a tumor based on shape or pixel intensities (histogram) with

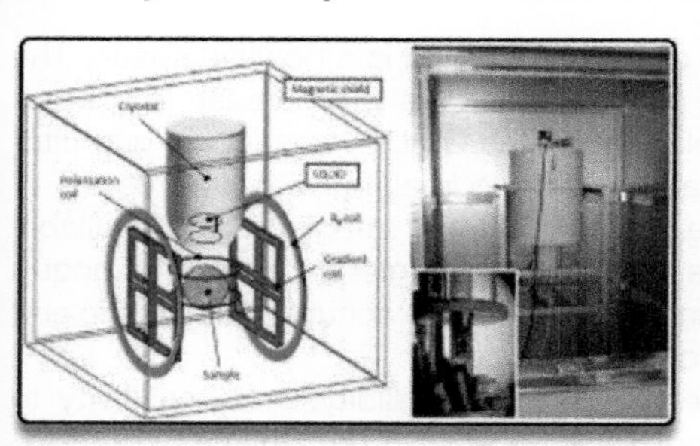

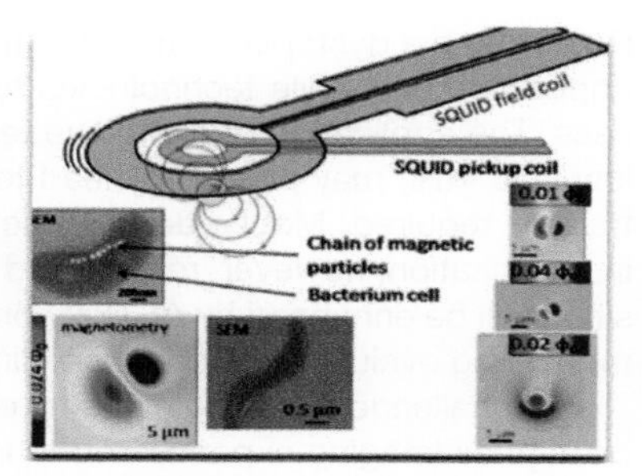

Fig. 5. Superconducting quantum interference devices (SQUIDs) and ultra low field MRI.

statistical machine learning models able to fit the data to potential imaging-based outcomes.[28] Fundamentally, the predefined feeders and traditional machine learning allow diagnosis, selection of abnormal tissue and assisting classification of that tissue.

Deep learning algorithms

One of the most exciting advances in AI research have led to deep learning algorithms that do not require the traditional explicit feature definitions and represent a different paradigm in machine learning. Convolutional neural networks comprise a series of layers that map image input to desired end points.[29,30] The abnormality is identified, extracted, selected, and then classified simultaneously during AI training. For the field of oncology in particular, deep machine learning algorithms assist in image characterization with segmentation, diagnosis of the image based on the classification abnormalities, staging of the image, and monitoring of the image.

Within the AI radiology paradigm, there are a number of functions that could potentially be augmented by AI implementation. The detection of abnormalities traditionally relies on a radiologist to use his or her experience and training to identify possible abnormalities, followed by intellectual processing to accept or reject the discovery. As computer methods advance, automated methods for the identification and processing of these predefined features—together known as computer-aided detection (CADe)—have been proposed.[31] Owing to the subhuman performance of traditional CADe technology, recent efforts have examined deep learning-based CADe techniques and early results show that using convolutional neural networks and deep learning algorithm CADe outperforms traditional CADe systems at low sensitivity while performing comparably at high sensitivity.[32]

The characterization of abnormalities is the second stage in the evolution of AI in radiology. Computer-based algorithms can be used to differentiate abnormal from normal tissue, inflamed from noninflamed tissue, with deep learning techniques able to learn from population-based abnormalities, applying a meticulous understanding of variations in anatomy, to provide enhanced characterization of normal from abnormal.[33]

Monitoring of disease is essential for the evaluation of treatment response. In rheumatology, as treatment becomes more effective and traditional clinical features become subclinical, this would include, for example, monitoring diminutive changes in synovitis, osteitis, erosions, and tenosynovitis as well as changes in the enthesis or sacroiliac joints. The process would encapsulate image registration where the diseased tissue is aligned across multiple time points, followed by an evaluation of metrics on time points using predefined protocols, allowing documentation and quantification of change.[34]

FUTURE PERSPECTIVES

Rather than a dystopian future, the future of mobile imaging is a positive space. The application of mobile technologies to the display of images will increase image access. The application of disruptive technology, such as CMUT transducers and ultra low field MRI, may potentially lead to greater access to imaging with lower levels of training required. Mobile devices increase the possibility of imaging being available in any location; however, remote and transfer of images for interpretation after acquisition will be enhanced by AI, likely providing rapid and more accurate diagnostic and monitoring evaluation to enhance clinical care.

The challenge for imaging is to ensure the reliability, validity, and sensitivity to change as imaging expands and to incorporate AI carefully. The meticulous assessment of new technology is the only way to ensure that mobile imaging remains a robust outcome measure, providing accurate information to guide clinicians and augment results in clinical trials.

REFERENCES

1. McKay FH, Cheng C, Wright A, et al. Evaluating mobile phone applications for health behaviour change: a systematic review [review]. J Telemed Telecare 2018;24(1):22–30.
2. Ventola CL. Mobile devices and apps for health care professionals: uses and benefits. P T 2014;39(5):356–64.
3. Thomairy NA, Mummaneni M, Alsalamah S, et al. Use of smartphones in hospitals. Health Care Manag (Frederick) 2015;34(4):297–307.
4. Silva LA, Costa C, Oliveira JL. DICOM relay over the cloud [review]. Int J Comput Assist Radiol Surg 2013;8(3):323–33.
5. Larobina M, Murino L. Medical image file formats. J Digit Imaging 2014;27(2): 200–6.
6. Graham RN, Perriss RW, Scarsbrook AF. DICOM demystified: a review of digital file formats and their use in radiological practice. Clin Radiol 2005;60(11): 1133–40.
7. Food and Drug Administration. Summary of safety and effectiveness MIM software December 2, 2011. 2011. Available at: https://www.accessdata.fda.gov/cdrh_dcs/pdf11/K112930.pdf. Accessed November 2, 2018.
8. Food and Drug Administration 2010 Department of Health and Human Services. Document control room K10342. 510(k) Summary of safety and effectiveness workstation OsiriX CF 807.92 Nov24, 2010. Available at: https://www.accessdata.fda.gov/cdrh_docs/pdf10/K103546.pdf. Accessed November 2, 2018.
9. Rosset A, Spadola L, Ratib O. OsiriX: an open-source software for navigating in multidimensional DICOM images. J Digit Imaging 2004;17(3):205–16 [review].
10. Möller I, Janta I, Backhaus M, et al. The 2017 EULAR standardised procedures for ultrasound imaging in rheumatology. Ann Rheum Dis 2017;76(12):1974–9.
11. Spiriev T, Nakov V, Laleva L, et al. OsiriX software as a preoperative planning tool in cranial neurosurgery: a step-by-step guide for neurosurgical residents. Surg Neurol Int 2017;8:241 [review].
12. Fortin M, Battié MC. Quantitative paraspinal muscle measurements: inter-software reliability and agreement using OsiriX and ImageJ. Phys Ther 2012;92(6):853–64.
13. Ariani A, Carotti M, Gutierrez M, et al. Utility of an open-source DICOM viewer software (OsiriX) to assess pulmonary fibrosis in systemic sclerosis: preliminary results. Rheumatol Int 2014;34(4):511–6.
14. D'Agostino MA, Schmidt WA. Ultrasound-guided injections in rheumatology: actual knowledge on efficacy and procedures. Best Pract Res Clin Rheumatol 2013;27(2):283–94.
15. Terslev L, Hammer HB, Torp-Pedersen S, et al. EFSUMB minimum training requirements for rheumatologists performing musculoskeletal ultrasound. Ultraschall Med 2013;34(5):475–7.
16. Food and Drug Administration. Summary of safety and effectiveness Poseidon Ultrasound System, Butterfly Inc. Sept. 6, 2017. 2018. Available at: https://www.accessdata.fda.gov/cdrh_docs/pdf16/K163510.pdf. Accessed November 2, 2018.
17. Khuri-Yakub BT, Oralkan O. Capacitive micromachined ultrasonic transducers for medical imaging and therapy. J Micromech Microeng 2011;21(5):54004–14.

18. Salim MS, Abd Malek MF, Heng RBW, et al. Capacitive micromachined ultrasonic transducers: technology and application. J Med Ultrasound 2012;20(1):8–31.
19. Ergun AS, Huang Y, Zhuang X, et al. Capacitive micromachined ultrasonic transducers: fabrication technology. IEEE Trans Ultrason Ferroelectr Freq Control 2005;52(12):2242–58.
20. Ostergaard M, Moller-Bisgard S. Optimal use of MRI in clinical trials, clinical care and clinical registries of patients with rheumatoid arthritis. Clin Exp Rheumatol 2014;32(Suppl 85):S17–22.
21. Bird P, Conaghan P, Ejbjerg B, et al. The development of the EULAR-OMERACT rheumatoid arthritis MRI reference image atlas [review]. Ann Rheum Dis 2005; 64(Suppl 1):i8–10.
22. Ostergaard M, McQueen F, Wiell C, et al. The OMERACT psoriatic arthritis magnetic resonance imaging scoring system (PsAMRIS): definitions of key pathologies, suggested MRI sequences, and preliminary scoring system for PsA hands. J Rheumatol 2009;36(8):1816–24.
23. Bird P, Ejbjerg B, Lassere M, et al. A multireader reliability study comparing conventional high-field magnetic resonance imaging with extremity low-field MRI in rheumatoid arthritis. J Rheumatol 2007;34(4):854–6.
24. United States Department of Defense. Special reports traumatic brain injury in service personnel 2017. Available at: https://dod.defense.gov. Accessed November 2, 2018.
25. Matlashov AN, Schultz LJ, Espy MA, et al. SQUIDs vs. induction coils for ultra-low field nuclear magnetic resonance: experimental and simulation comparison. IEEE Trans Appl Supercond 2011;21(3):465–8.
26. Espy M, Matlashov A, Volegov P. SQUID-detected ultra-low field MRI. J Magn Reson 2013;228:1–15.
27. Sandin HJ, Volegov PL, Espy MA, et al. Noise modeling from conductive shields using Kirchhoff equations. IEEE Trans Appl Supercond 2010;21(3):489–92.
28. Nagaraj S, Rao GN, Koteswararao K. The role of pattern recognition in computer-aided diagnosis and computer- aided detection in medical imaging: a clinical validation. Int J Comput Appl 2010;8:18–22.
29. Tajbakhsh N, Shin JY, Gurudu SR, et al. Convolutional neural networks for medical image analysis: full training or fine tuning? IEEE Trans Med Imaging 2016;35(5): 1299–312.
30. Chartrand G, Cheng PM, Vorontsov E, et al. Deep learning: a primer for radiologists [review]. Radiographics 2017;37(7):2113–31.
31. Firmino M, Angelo G, Morais H, et al. Computer-aided detection (CADe) and diagnosis (CADx) system for lung cancer with likelihood of malignancy. Biomed Eng Online 2016;15:2.
32. Shin HC, Roth HR, Gao M, et al. Deep convolutional neural networks for computer-aided detection: CNN architectures, dataset characteristics and transfer learning. IEEE Trans Med Imaging 2016;35(5):1285–98.
33. Giannini V, Mazzetti S, Vignati A, et al. A fully automatic computer aided diagnosis system for peripheral zone prostate cancer detection using multi- parametric magnetic resonance imaging. Comput Med Imaging Graph 2015;46:219–26.
34. Patriarche JW, Erickson BJ. Part 1. Automated change detection and characterization in serial MR studies of brain- tumor patients. J Digit Imaging 2007;20: 203–22.

Project ECHO

Telehealth to Expand Capacity to Deliver Best Practice Medical Care

E. Michael Lewiecki, MD[a,*], Rachelle Rochelle, MPA[b]

KEYWORDS

• ECHO • TeleECHO • Telehealth • Telemedicine • Osteoporosis • Treatment

KEY POINTS

- Project ECHO (Extension for Community Healthcare Outcomes) is a model of interactive ongoing case-based learning using videoconferencing technology to educate health care professionals located anywhere there is an Internet connection.
- ECHO has been shown to elevate the level of knowledge of primary care providers in underserved communities to provide specialty level care for chronic complex diseases.
- ECHO allows patients to receive better care, closer to home, with greater convenience and lower cost than referral to a specialty center.
- ECHO aims to increase capacity to deliver best practice medical care worldwide.

BACKGROUND

There is a global shortage and maldistribution of health care professionals that limits access to essential medical services, especially in rural areas. The World Health Organization (WHO) reports that countries at all levels of socioeconomic development have difficulties in education, deployment, retention, and performance of the health care workforce.[1] The WHO goes on to state there is a need to modify and correct the configuration and supply of physician generalists and specialists, advanced

Disclosure Statement: In the past year, E.M. Lewiecki has received institutional grant or research support from Radius, Amgen, PFEnex, and Mereo; he has served on scientific advisory boards or consulted for Amgen, Radius, Alexion, Ultragenyx, Sandoz, and Celltrion; he serves on the speakers' bureau for Radius and Alexion; he is a board member of the National Osteoporosis Foundation, International Society for Clinical Densitometry, and Osteoporosis Foundation of New Mexico. R. Rochelle has nothing to disclose. No funding was received for development, writing, or revising this article.
[a] New Mexico Clinical Research & Osteoporosis Center, 300 Oak Street NE, Albuquerque, NM 87106, USA; [b] Project ECHO, University of New Mexico Health Sciences Center, 1650 University Boulevard NE Albuquerque, NM 87102, USA
* Corresponding author.
E-mail address: mlewiecki@gmail.com

Rheum Dis Clin N Am 45 (2019) 303–314
https://doi.org/10.1016/j.rdc.2019.01.003
rheumatic.theclinics.com

practitioners (eg, nurse practitioners, physician assistants), and community health workers, recommending that health care systems develop a team-based primary care approach by fully harnessing the potential of technological innovation.[1] Physician supply and demand in the United States has been assessed in a report prepared for the Association of American Medical Colleges.[2] It was projected that the demand for physicians will continue to grow faster than the supply, with a projected shortfall of primary care physicians between 7300 and 43,100, and projected shortfalls of nonprimary care specialties between 33,500 and 61,800 by 2030. Among the specialists in short supply are rheumatologists and endocrinologists.

The 2015 Workforce Study of Rheumatology Specialists in the United States described trends and projected supply and demand for physicians, nurse practitioners, and physician assistants from 2015 to 2030 using primary and secondary data sources.[3] The findings were influenced by major demographic and geographic shifts that included baby-boomer retirements, an aging population, increase of part-time providers, and increasing demand for adult rheumatology care. It was estimated that demand exceeded supply of clinical full-time equivalents (FTEs) by 12.9% in 2015 and will increase to 102% by 2030. There was an imbalance of workforce retirement in excess of those entering the workforce and maldistribution of the workforce according to region of the country, with the 2015 ratio of adult rheumatology providers per 100,000 patients ranging from 3.07 in the Northeast (projected to decrease to 1.61 by 2025) to 1.28 in the Southwest (projected to decrease to 0.64 by 2025). Telemedicine, telehealth, and telerheumatology were listed as potential strategies to improve timely access to rheumatology care in underserved communities.

The Endocrine Society commissioned an Endocrinology Workforce Analysis by the Lewin Group to estimate current and projected workforce for clinical endocrinology care. It was concluded that there are too few adult endocrinologists to meet current and future demand, with an excess demand gap of about 1484 FTEs in 2015 and 1344 FTEs projected by 2025.[4] The current demand for the services of endocrinologists is driven by diabetes mellitus, which represents 46.1% of coded visits.[4] As with rheumatologists, there was an imbalance between annual entrants into adult endocrinology and attrition due to retirement and other factors, as well as maldistribution, with a higher concentration of endocrinologists in New England and Middle Atlantic regions and relative scarcity in other regions of the United States. Again, telemedicine was identified as a means to disseminate information about best practices and reduce the gap between supply and demand.

TELEMEDICINE AND TELEHEALTH

There are no universally accepted definitions for telemedicine and telehealth. Tele- is a form meaning distant or at a distance. One of the first uses of modern technology for communicating medical information was by Willem Einthoven, a Dutch physician and physiologist, in 1905. He developed the first electrocardiograph in his laboratory in Leiden, Netherlands, and used a string galvanometer and telephone wires to transmit cardiac signals between his laboratory and a hospital 1.5 km away.[5] He was awarded the Nobel Prize in Medicine in 1924 for his discovery of the electrocardiograph. The term telemedicine began to appear in the medical literature in the 1970s, when it was used to describe a 2-way audiovisual microwave circuit that connected physicians at Massachusetts General Hospital with patients at Logan International Airport Medical Station 2.7 miles away.[6] There are now many highly sophisticated electronic audiovisual communication systems that transmit and receive a vast range of information with broad applications for health care.

When tele- is applied to health care, the words telemedicine and telehealth are sometimes used interchangeably to mean that health information is exchanged electronically from 1 location to another. Others have used telehealth as an all-encompassing term that includes telemedicine. Recent reviews have highlighted numerous complexities of terminology and applications to health care.[7,8] The Office for the Advancement of Telehealth at the US Health Resources & Services Administration broadly defines telehealth as "the use of electronic information and telecommunication technologies to support and promote long-distance clinical health care, patient and professional health-related education, public health and health administration."[9] Operationally, telemedicine typically implies the delivery of diagnostic or therapeutic medical services at a distance, whereas telehealth often refers to health education at a distance. These definitions are used in this article. When telemedicine is applied for 1 health care professional or a team of health care professionals to care for 1 patient located at a distance, it can be a great benefit for the patient but does not expand the capacity to deliver health care. From a health system viewpoint, it is simply substituting a patient located remotely for 1 who might have been seen in the clinic. When telehealth is applied to the education of many health care professionals at a distance, it has the potential to serve as a force multiplier to improve the care of many patients located wherever the participant health care professionals are located.

This article describes the development and progress of Project ECHO (Extension for Community Healthcare Outcomes), a strategy of case-based learning with videoconferencing (**Table 1**), highlighting osteoporosis as the principal disease model. Although there is no single specialty with exclusive rights to care for osteoporosis, ECHO has relevance for primary care providers, who care for most patients with osteoporosis,

Table 1
Comparison of ECHO with other forms of online health care and online learning

Features	TeleECHO	Telehealth	Telemedicine	Webinar
Hub and spoke model	✓	✓	—	✓
Videoconferencing	✓	✓	✓	✓
Addresses underserved populations	✓	✓	✓	—
Direct doctor–patient relationship	—	—	✓	—
Deidentified patients	✓	✓	—	—
Remote patient monitoring	—	—	✓	—
Interactive case-based learning	✓	✓	—	—
Oral presentations	✓	✓	—	✓
CME credit	✓	✓	✓	✓
Reimbursement for patient care (CPT codes)	—	—	✓	—
Predominately lecture format	—	—	—	✓
Development of subspecialty expertise over time	✓	—	—	—
Demonopolization of specialty knowledge	✓	—	—	—

TeleECHO has many features of telehealth, with the capacity for participants to develop subspecialty expertise over time[10,11] by demonopolizing specialty knowledge.[38] Telemedicine usually involves 1 physician caring for 1 patient at a distance. A Webinar is typically a lecture online with limited opportunity for interactive discussions and ongoing learning.

Abbreviation: CPT, current procedural terminology.

Courtesy of Project ECHO, University of New Mexico Health Sciences Center, Albuquerque, NM.

and rheumatologists and endocrinologists, who are often perceived as having special expertise in the care of osteoporosis.

PROJECT EXTENSION FOR COMMUNITY HEALTHCARE OUTCOMES

The prototype Project ECHO program for remote learning began in 2003, at the University of New Mexico (UNM) Health Sciences Center in Albuquerque, New Mexico, USA. It was started by an academic gastroenterologist because of a large treatment gap for the care of chronic hepatitis C. At that time in New Mexico there were approximately 34,000 patients diagnosed with hepatitis C but fewer than 1600 receiving treatment.[10] Lack of treatment was attributed to factors that included patients living large distances from specialists at the UNM gastroenterology (GI) clinic in Albuquerque, too few specialists at the clinic, long wait times for appointments, time and money needed for travel, primary providers lacking expertise in treating hepatitis C, treatment side effects, and cultural issues. The ECHO model (**Fig. 1**) used videoconferencing with a hub-and-spoke system that linked a team of experts at a hub (training center) at the university with primary care providers at spokes (community clinics) in rural New Mexico. Each session included a brief presentation on a topic of interest. Learning also occurred through real-time case-based discussions of deidentified patients presented by the participants. Because the discussions provided the basis for learning but did not constitute a consultation or direct patient care, there were no concerns regarding professional liability.

The outcomes of the ECHO intervention were evaluated with a prospective cohort study comparing treatment of hepatitis C at UNM with treatment by primary care physicians at 21 ECHO sites located in rural communities and prisons in New Mexico.[11] The primary endpoint was sustained virologic response. An analysis of outcomes for 407 patients managed by participants at the ECHO sites showed a sustained virologic response (58.2% of patients) that was similar to patients treated at the UNM GI clinic (57.5% of patients, $P = 0.89$). Serious adverse events were reported in 6.9% of patients at the ECHO sites compared with 13.7% of patients at the UNM clinic. This study demonstrated that the ECHO model could be implemented in rural and underserved communities to improve the care of patients with hepatitis C. These patients, who were receiving no treatment before ECHO, were treated at least as well as those treated at the GI clinic after the ECHO intervention. These findings supported continued use of ECHO for hepatitis C and further development of ECHO to improve clinical outcomes for other chronic complex diseases with effective treatments that are underutilized. The ECHO Project was subsequently established at UNM with a mission to expand capacity to safely and effectively treat chronic, common, complex conditions in rural and underserved areas. The ECHO model of learning has since been adapted for many disease states, including the use of the model with nonmedical education interventions, throughout the United States and globally.[12–21]

Project ECHO now has more than 250 hubs for more than 100 diseases and conditions with more than 550 programs in 33 countries.[22] It continues to expand, with a goal of touching the lives of 1 billion people by 2025. There are currently 6 rheumatology programs and 17 endocrinology or diabetes programs, with more expected to follow.

ECHO is a force multiplier that expands capacity to deliver best practice medical care through networks for sharing knowledge. Because each ECHO participant manages many patients, more patients will have better care, closer to home, with greater convenience, and lower cost than referral to a specialty center. ECHO can be scaled to any level through replication (development of more ECHO hubs), allowing it to function

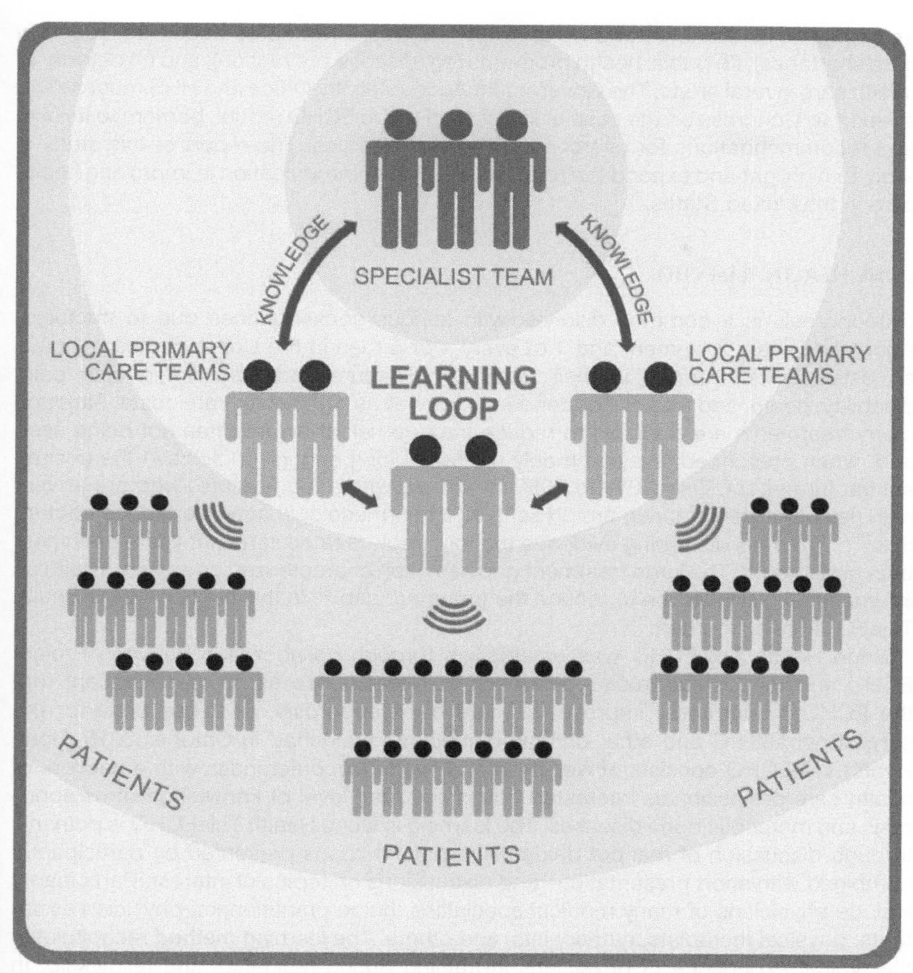

Fig. 1. ECHO model of learning. A faculty team uses videoconferencing to connect with individuals and teams of health care professionals to share knowledge of best practice care. Learning is primarily through discussion of real but deidentified case presentations. Each participant cares for many patients who may benefit from the knowledge attained. (*Courtesy of* Project ECHO, University of New Mexico Health Sciences Center, Albuquerque, NM. © Project ECHO. 2018; with permission.)

in the right time zone, at convenient times, and using the appropriate language for its participants. ECHO can be implemented anywhere there is electronic access to connect the participants. After initial training on fidelity to the ECHO model, provided at no cost by Project ECHO, most ECHO hubs operate independently.

The US government has recognized, with recent legislation, the potential of using telecommunications to educate health care professionals. The Expanding Capacity for Health Outcomes Act (ECHO Act)[23] was signed by President Obama in December 2016. The ECHO Act tasks the Secretary of the Department of Health and Human Services (HHS) to study the infrastructure of Project ECHO and examine its effects in 4 areas: (1) mental health and substance use disorders, chronic conditions, maternal and pediatric health, and palliative care; (2) health care workforce issues (eg, specialty care shortages); (3) public health programs (eg, disease prevention); and (4) delivery of health care in rural areas. The Government Accountability Office and HHS must deliver a report to Congress on the ease of integration of the ECHO model, barriers to its use, and recommendations for overcoming those challenges. The report of this study is likely to highlight and expand the role of electronic communication in improving health care in the United States.[24]

BONE HEALTH TeleECHO

Osteoporosis is a common disorder with serious consequences due to fractures. About 1 of every 2 women, and 1 of every 4 or 5 men in the United States will have an osteoporotic fracture in their lifetime.[25] Fractures are associated with pain, disability, death, and loss of independence, as well as high health care costs. Although many treatments are available to reduce fracture risk, they are often not being used and, when prescribed, are commonly not taken long enough to achieve the desired antifracture effect. Only 10% to 20% of women with a hip fracture, who are at very high risk of future fractures, are prescribed a pharmacologic agent to reduce fracture risk.[26,27] There is disturbing evidence that hip fracture rates in recent years are higher than projected.[28] The large treatment gap has been characterized as a crisis,[29] with an international call to action to reduce the treatment gap.[30] In this context, Bone Health TeleECHO has emerged.[31]

Bone Health TeleECHO was established through collaboration between Project ECHO and the Osteoporosis Foundation of New Mexico as proof-of-concept that the ECHO model could improve the care of osteoporosis, as it has done for the care of hepatitis C and other chronic conditions. Launched in October 2015, Bone Health TeleECHO consists of weekly interactive videoconferences with a network of health care professionals interested advancing their level of knowledge of osteoporosis and metabolic bone diseases. The learning in Bone Health TeleECHO is primarily through discussion of real but deidentified patient cases presented by participants, combined with short presentations and discussions on topics of interest. Participants include physicians of many medical specialties, nurse practitioners, physician assistants, physical therapists, nutritionists, and others. The learning method recapitulates the typical experience of physicians-in-training during residency and fellowship, in which interactive case-based discussions are the main source of acquiring new knowledge. The aims of Bone Health TeleECHO are to improve the skeletal care of patients of the participants and serve as a model for replication in other states and countries.[31–33]

Each weekly Bone Health TeleECHO session is 75 minutes in duration. Participants may log in for every session or intermittently, according to the level of interest. Some participate as desired for presenting a case or for a particular presentation. Funding is provided through grants received by Project ECHO at UNM. Staff support includes a coordinator engaged for about 10 hours for each TeleECHO session to assist with all logistical aspects, including scheduling and continuing medical education (CME) evaluations, as well as interfacing with faculty, participants, and speakers. The TeleECHO program is physically located in a videoconferencing room at the hub, with some faculty and participants present; other participants are located virtually, anywhere there is an Internet connection. An information technology specialist is also on site, which is helpful in allowing the TeleECHO session moderator to focus on facilitating the discussions without unnecessary distractions from technical issues. Faculty members receive no direct compensation. No-cost CME credits are provided for TeleECHO participants by UNM. Presentations are recorded and archived online; these are available for viewing by registered ECHO participants who might have missed a session or want to view the presentations again. The recordings are also shared with other TeleECHO programs that have an interest in presenting the same topic.

THREE-YEAR EXPERIENCE OF BONE HEALTH TeleECHO

Bone Health TeleECHO was launched on October 5, 2015. Demographic data on participants are collected through online registrations. ECHO staff monitor attendance at each weekly TeleECHO session. Over the first 36 months, 145 videoconferencing sessions were held, with 487 individuals registering to participate, and 358 attending at least once. Average attendance for each session increased from 13 in 2015 to 42 in 2018. Physicians constituted 42% of participants, with the most common specialties being endocrinology, rheumatology, and orthopedics; advanced practice providers represented 23% of participants, with the remainder composed of a variety of medical disciplines, including physical therapy and occupational therapy. Participants were located across a large geographic area (**Fig. 2**), with 25% in New Mexico, 60% located in 40 other states, 3% from 9 other countries (Canada, Mexico, United Kingdom, Ireland, Spain, Chile, Brazil, Trinidad and Tobago, and Russia), and 12% unknown. In the first 36 months of Bone Health TeleECHO, 160 patient cases were presented and discussed, and more than 1682 hours of no-cost CME were provided.

Outcomes were assessed with a blinded self-efficacy questionnaire administered online after 10 months of Bone Health TeleECHO (**Fig. 3**).[34] Briefly, participants were asked to rate their self-confidence in 20 domains of osteoporosis care before and after the ECHO intervention, with a rating scale of 0 to 7 (7 is highest). Effect

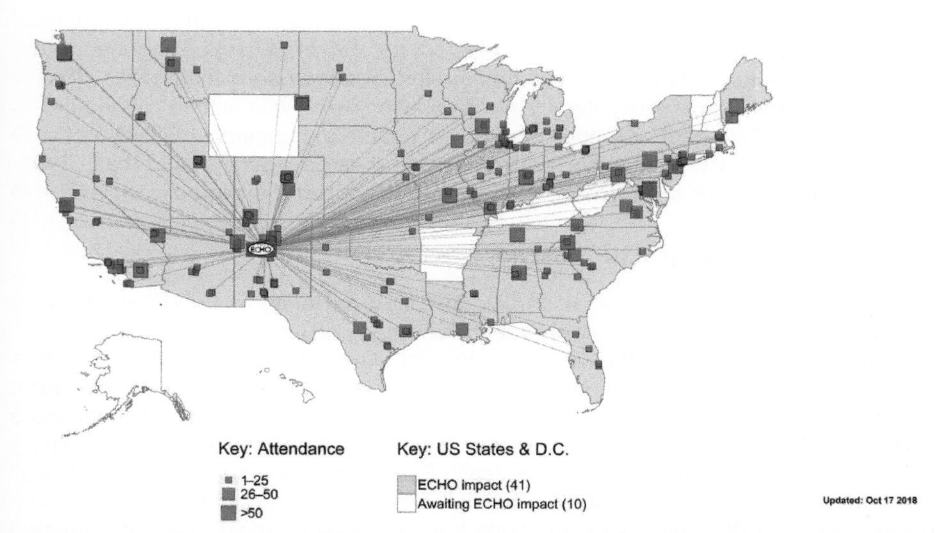

Fig. 2. Bone Health TeleECHO participant locations. This map of the United States illustrates the hub and spoke network (36-month data) that is a feature of the ECHO model of learning. There have also been participants from 9 other countries not included on this map. Other Bone Health TeleECHO hubs have been established in Grand Blanc, Michigan; Washington, DC; and Galway, Ireland. More hubs are expected soon. (*Courtesy of* Project ECHO, University of New Mexico Health Sciences Center, Albuquerque, NM. © Project ECHO. 2018; with permission.)

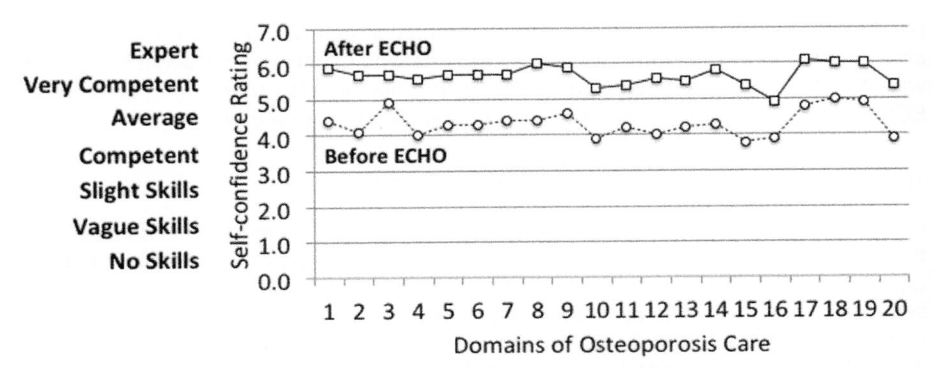

Fig. 3. Bone Health TeleECHO outcomes assessment. There were significant improvement ($P = .005$) in self-confidence in 20 different domains of osteoporosis care for health care professionals who have participated more than 10 teleECHO clinics. (*Adapted from* Lewiecki EM, Rochelle R, Bouchonville MF, et al. Leveraging scarce resources with bone health Tele-ECHO to improve the care of osteoporosis. J Endocr Soc 2017;1(12):1428–34).

size was classified according to the method of Cohen[35] and Sawilowsky[36] (0.2 = small, 0.5 = medium, 0.8 = large, 1.20 = very large effect size). There was a statistically significant overall improvement in confidence of caring for osteoporosis patients with an effect size of 1.18 ($P = .005$). Patient-level outcomes data would be preferable to self-efficacy but far more difficult to obtain. The ultimate desired outcome from the ECHO intervention is greater reduction in fracture risk for patients of participants. However, it is likely that as competency in osteoporosis care improves, the patient mix will evolve to include more patients at higher risk of fracture, therefore confounding interpretation of fracture data. Potential surrogates for better osteoporosis care with future studies might be number of bone density tests obtained, number of patients diagnosed with osteoporosis, and number of prescriptions for osteoporosis medications filled, assessed by analysis of health care claims databases linked with unique blinded provider identifiers. Comparator groups could be the same data points of ECHO participants before the ECHO intervention or similar health care providers without the ECHO intervention. Strategies for such an outcomes study are being explored.

REPLICATION OF BONE HEALTH TeleECHO

The progressive increase in levels of participation in Bone Health TeleECHO and favorable findings of the outcomes measurements have fostered interest in development of more Bone Health hubs in other locations. Project ECHO staff includes a team dedicated to facilitating the replication of ECHO worldwide. Monthly no-cost trainings for starting an ECHO program are conducted at UNM, typically with about 100 attendees from the United States and abroad. For those not able to attend, limited ECHO training is available online. All aspects of Bone Health ECHO, including curriculum, archived presentations, and case-presentation templates, are shared with others who wish to develop similar ECHO programs. Although it is not required, most ECHO programs use Zoom software[37] as the teleconferencing platform. Zoom is available to Project ECHO partners at no cost. Every 3 months, a collaborative videoconference is held for those who have already replicated Bone Health TeleECHO, and those who are considering doing so. The purpose is to make all aware of resources that are available, to share successes and challenges in operating an ECHO program, and provide assistance in developing and maintaining ECHO.

Other Bone Health TeleECHO programs have been launched, a hub in the state of Michigan and another in Washington, DC, with a focus on fracture liaison service coordinators, and a fourth in Galway, Ireland. More replications are expected in the near future.

LESSONS LEARNED AFTER 3 YEARS OF BONE HEALTH TeleECHO

While remaining true to the model of interactive case-based learning, each hub and the TeleECHO program it provides evolves with a flavor of its own that depends on factors that include the location, needs of the participants, the interests of the faculty, the disease state, and numerous other local circumstances. The experience of Bone Health TeleECHO is described here. Based on the first TeleECHO program devoted to the treatment of chronic hepatitis C, it was expected that Bone Health TeleECHO would predominantly involve primary care providers in rural New Mexico who were professionally isolated. The experience with Bone Health TeleECHO was profoundly different.

Primary Care Providers

Many primary care physicians and advanced practice providers have participated. However, the most common physician attendees are from the following specialties: endocrinology, rheumatology, and orthopedics. Many other medical disciplines have also taken part, including physical therapists, occupational therapists, and nutritionists, all of whom contribute to the learning experience by viewing clinical conditions through a different lens.

Rural Locations

Some participants are in rural locations. However, many are in urban areas. The desire to acquire a higher level on knowledge about osteoporosis and metabolic bone disease does not seem to be determined by geography. Underserved communities can be urban as well as rural.

Professional Isolation

Primary care providers in rural locations are not the only health care professionals who are professionally isolated. It has been surprising to learn that health care professionals at any location (rural or urban), any specialty (primary care or specialty), any practice setting (private practice or academic), and any baseline level of knowledge (beginner or advanced) can enjoy and benefit from the collegial method of learning with the ECHO model.

OPPORTUNITIES, CHALLENGES, AND LIMITATIONS

Project ECHO offers a vast array of support services to aid in the development of an ECHO hub, which may then provide 1 or more programs according to needs and local resources. Anyone interested in starting an ECHO hub can benefit from the experience of others in the form of collaboration and shared information on the ECHO Web site at https://echo.unm.edu/. There are staff members devoted to replication, archived files that are shared with ECHO partners, examples of curricula, templates for case presentations, online and in-person mentoring, assistance in obtaining CME, guidance for obtaining funding, and more, most of which is at no cost.

Starting an ECHO hub requires at least 1 passionate individual with leadership skills, dedicated time, and a high level of motivation to make a difference in educating health care professionals. The designated director and moderator should be assigned the task of moving the process forward. A hub faculty team must be assembled; this team can be located at the physical location of the ECHO hub or anywhere else there is an Internet connection. A program coordinator is needed to facilitate the many logistics of planning, scheduling the sessions, CME, and outcomes measurements. Availability of technical support is helpful but not required; often, if program coordinators are comfortable with technology, they can also assist with this role. A videoconferencing center is ideal for a physical hub; this is commonly available, often at no cost, from a university, hospital, or institution, which may provide information technology assistance as well. Funding must be obtained locally or through sources such as private and public grants or governmental agencies. Ultimately, payers of medical services may see the benefit of ECHO in terms of reducing costs (eg, fewer hospitalizations, fewer consultations with specialists) and be willing to support ECHO programs.

Because interactive case-based learning is a key feature of ECHO, there may be diminishing educational benefits as a single ECHO program becomes very large. The optimal number of participants for ECHO is uncertain and may vary according to the disease state and style of the moderator. To act as a highly effective force multiplier and truly expand global capacity to deliver best practice medical care, ECHO for each disease state must be replicated many times over. Because the ECHO model can be scaled to any level, this is achievable.

FUTURE DIRECTIONS

The delivery of medical care has become more complex and more expensive worldwide. Health care professionals everywhere struggle with demands on their time and services. The inconvenience and cost of travel to medical congresses limits the effectiveness in reaching providers of medical services. The lecture format of medical education is arguably less likely to result in changes in practice patterns than learning by discussion of patient cases. Private foundations and governments are increasingly turning to technologies such as videoconferencing to improve health care delivery. The ECHO model of learning is expected to continue to expand, with applications for many aspects of health care and other disciplines.

SUMMARY

ECHO is an educational model that provides ongoing mentoring of health care professionals through videoconferencing with case-based interactive learning, brief oral presentations, and sharing of best practices. It has been shown to be effective in elevating the level of knowledge of health care professionals in rural and underserved areas to deliver subspecialty care for patients closer to home with greater convenience and lower cost than referral to a specialty center. The experience of Bone Health TeleECHO provides proof-of-concept that this model of learning can be replicated in many locations worldwide to expand capacity to deliver best practice medical care worldwide.

REFERENCES

1. World Health Organization. Global strategy on human resources for health: workforce 2030 2016. Available at: http://www.who.int/hrh/resources/global_strategy_workforce2030_14_print.pdf?ua=1. Accessed October 6, 2018.
2. IHS Markit. The complexities of physician supply and demand: projections from 2015 to 2030 2017. Available at: https://aamc-black.global.ssl.fastly.net/production/media/filer_public/a5/c3/a5c3d565-14ec-48fb-974b-99fafaeecb00/aamc_projections_update_2017.pdf. Accessed October 6, 2018.

3. Battafarano DF, Ditmyer M, Bolster MB, et al. 2015 American College of Rheumatology Workforce Study: supply and demand projections of adult rheumatology workforce, 2015-2030. Arthritis Care Res (Hoboken) 2018;70(4):617–26.
4. Vigersky RA, Fish L, Hogan P, et al. The clinical endocrinology workforce: current status and future projections of supply and demand. J Clin Endocrinol Metab 2014;99(9):3112–21.
5. Einthoven W. The telecardiogram. Am Heart J 1957;53(4):163–211.
6. Murphy RL Jr, Bird KT. Telediagnosis: a new community health resource. Observations on the feasibility of telediagnosis based on 1000 patient transactions. Am J Public Health 1974;64(2):113–9.
7. Waller M, Stotler C. Telemedicine: a Primer. Curr Allergy Asthma Rep 2018; 18(10):54.
8. Kvedar J, Coye MJ, Everett W. Connected health: a review of technologies and strategies to improve patient care with telemedicine and telehealth. Health Aff (Millwood) 2014;33(2):194–9.
9. Health Resources & Services Administration. Telehealth programs. Available at: https://www.hrsa.gov/rural-health/telehealth/index.html. Accessed October 6, 2018.
10. Arora S, Kalishman S, Dion D, et al. Partnering urban academic medical centers and rural primary care clinicians to provide complex chronic disease care. Health Aff (Millwood) 2011;30(6):1176–84.
11. Arora S, Thornton K, Murata G, et al. Outcomes of treatment for hepatitis C virus infection by primary care providers. N Engl J Med 2011;364(23):2199–207.
12. Dubin RE, Flannery J, Taenzer P, et al. ECHO Ontario chronic pain & opioid stewardship: providing access and building capacity for primary care providers in underserviced, rural, and remote communities. Stud Health Technol Inform 2015;209:15–22.
13. Kauth MR, Shipherd JC, Lindsay JA, et al. Teleconsultation and training of VHA providers on transgender care: implementation of a multisite hub system. Telemed J E Health 2015;21(12):1012–8.
14. Katzman JG, Comerci G Jr, Boyle JF, et al. Innovative telementoring for pain management: project ECHO pain. J Contin Educ Health Prof 2014;34(1):68–75.
15. Mitruka K, Thornton K, Cusick S, et al. Expanding primary care capacity to treat hepatitis C virus infection through an evidence-based care model–Arizona and Utah, 2012-2014. MMWR Morb Mortal Wkly Rep 2014;63(18):393–8.
16. Scott JD, Unruh KT, Catlin MC, et al. Project ECHO: a model for complex, chronic care in the Pacific Northwest region of the United States. J Telemed Telecare 2012;18(8):481–4.
17. Lewiecki EM, Bilezikian JP, Carey JJ, et al. Proceedings of the 2017 Santa Fe bone symposium: insights and emerging concepts in the management of osteoporosis. J Clin Densitom 2018;21(1):3–21.
18. Bennett KA, Ong T, Verrall AM, et al. Project ECHO-geriatrics: training future primary care providers to meet the needs of older adults. J Grad Med Educ 2018; 10(3):311–5.
19. Hager B, Hasselberg M, Arzubi E, et al. Leveraging behavioral health expertise: practices and potential of the project ECHO approach to virtually integrating care in underserved areas. Psychiatr Serv 2018;69(4):366–9.
20. Carlin L, Zhao J, Dubin R, et al. Project ECHO telementoring intervention for managing chronic pain in primary care: insights from a qualitative study. Pain Med 2018;19(6):1140–6.

21. Sockalingam S, Arena A, Serhal E, et al. Building provincial mental health capacity in primary care: an evaluation of a project ECHO mental health program. Acad Psychiatry 2018;42(4):451–7.
22. Project ECHO. ECHO hubs and superhubs: global 2018. Available at: https://echo.unm.edu/locations-2/echo-hubs-superhubs-global/. Accessed October 14, 2018.
23. www.GovTrack.us. S. 2873(114th): ECHO Act. (May 29, 2017). Available at: https://www.govtrack.us/congress/bills/114/s2873. Accessed August 3, 2017.
24. Goerlich C. Congress passed the ECHO Act—what does this mean for telehealth?. 2016. Available at: https://www.advisory.com/research/market-innovation-center/the-growth-channel/2016/12/telehealth-echo. Accessed October 6, 2018.
25. Cosman F, de Beur SJ, LeBoff MS, et al. Clinician's guide to prevention and treatment of osteoporosis. Osteoporos Int 2014;25(10):2359–81.
26. Solomon DH, Johnston SS, Boytsov NN, et al. Osteoporosis medication use after hip fracture in U.S. patients between 2002 and 2011. J Bone Miner Res 2014;29(9):1929–37.
27. Gillespie CW, Morin PE. Osteoporosis-related health services utilization following first hip fracture among a cohort of privately-insured women in the United States, 2008-2014: an observational study. J Bone Miner Res 2017;32(5):1052–61.
28. Lewiecki EM, Wright NC, Curtis JR, et al. Hip fracture trends in the United States, 2002 to 2015. Osteoporos Int 2018;29(3):717–22.
29. Khosla S, Shane E. A crisis in the treatment of osteoporosis. J Bone Miner Res 2016;31(8):1485–7.
30. American Society for Bone and Mineral Research. Call to action to address the crisis in the treatment of osteoporosis 2016. Available at: https://www.asbmr.org/call-to-action.aspx. Accessed January 11, 2017.
31. Lewiecki EM, Boyle JF, Arora S, et al. Telementoring: a novel approach to reducing the osteoporosis treatment gap. Osteoporos Int 2017;28(1):407–11.
32. Lewiecki EM. Bone Health TeleECHO for orthopedists and rheumatologists. Ortho Rheum Open Access 2017;7(4):555716. Available at: https://juniperpublishers.com/oroaj/pdf/OROAJ.MS.ID.555716.pdf. Accessed February 14, 2019.
33. Lewiecki EM, Bouchonville MF 2nd, Chafey DH, et al. Bone Health ECHO: telementoring to improve osteoporosis care. Womens Health (Lond) 2016;12(1):79–81.
34. Lewiecki EM, Rochelle R, Bouchonville MF 2nd, et al. Leveraging scarce resources with bone health TeleECHO to improve the care of osteoporosis. J Endocr Soc 2017;1(12):1428–34.
35. Cohen J. Statistical power analysis for the behavioral sciences. 2nd edition. Hillsdale (NJ): L. Erlbaum Associates; 1988.
36. Sawilowsky S. New effect size rules of thumb. J Mod Appl Stat Methods 2009;8(2):467–74.
37. Zoom. The cloud meeting company. Available at: https://operative.zoom.us/. Accessed October 27, 2018.
38. Arora S, Thornton K, Komaromy M, et al. Demonopolizing medical knowledge. Acad Med 2014;89(1):30–2.

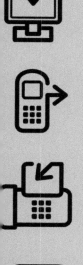

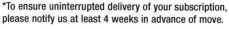

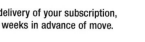

Printed and bound by CPI Group (UK) Ltd, Croydon, CR0 4YY

Printed and bound by CPI Group (UK) Ltd, Croydon, CR0 4YY
08/05/2025
01864745-0008